TOTAL
Reflexology

TOTAL
Reflexology

The Reflex Points for Physical, Emotional, and Psychological Healing

Martine Faure-Alderson, D.O.

Translated by Jon E. Graham

Healing Arts Press
Rochester, Vermont

Healing Arts Press
One Park Street
Rochester, Vermont 05767
www.HealingArtsPress.com

Healing Arts Press is a division of Inner Traditions International

Originally published in French under the title *Réflexologie thérapie totale: Du réflexe à la conscience* by Guy
    Trédaniel Éditeur
First U.S. edition published in 2008 by Healing Arts Press

*Note to the reader: This book is intended as an informational guide. The remedies, approaches, and techniques
described herein are meant to supplement, and not to be a substitute for, professional medical care or treatment. They should not be used to treat a serious ailment without prior consultation with a qualified health care
professional.*

Library of Congress Cataloging-in-Publication Data
Faure-Alderson, Martine.
  [Réflexologie thérapie totale. English]
  Total reflexology : the reflex points for physical, emotional, and psychological healing / Martine Faure-
Alderson ; translated by Jon E. Graham.
    p. ; cm.
  Includes bibliographical references and index.
  ISBN 978-1-59477-247-4 (pbk.) — ISBN 978-1-59477-261-0 (hardcover)
  1. Reflexology (Therapy) 2. Foot—Massage. I. Title.
  [DNLM: 1. Massage—methods. 2. Foot. WB 537 F265r 2008a]
  RM723.R43F3813 2008
  615.8'22—dc22

                                                                                            2008025108

Printed and bound in India by Replika Press Pvt. Ltd.

10 9 8 7 6 5 4 3 2 1

Text design and layout by Priscilla Baker
This book was typeset in Minion with Perpetua and Helvetica Neue used as display typefaces

Those wishing to contact the author, may write to her at
    martinefa@craniosacralreflexologyinstitute.com
To find out about the author's training program in Total Reflexology Therapy visit
    www.craniosacralreflexologyinstitute.com

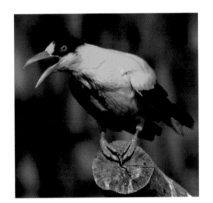

MONKEY BUSINESS

My papa is tall
He wears a mustache
My mama is pretty
She has large eyelashes
of sky blue.

My buddy is Lulu
My best friend is Delphine
She is sweet through and through
Her cheeks are full of
Honey!

When I get bigger
And I own some boots
I will jump in the puddles
And walk in lion's
Poop!

Papa will give me his look,
He will stare right at me,
Right straight into my little eyes
While mama will make little shrieks
Like a mouse!

And when they're not around
Me and my buddy Lulu
And her little sister Denise
We can get into all the monkey business
we want!

We can give the dog a haircut
Boil soap
Stick the cat in the piano
And play la Marseillaise
In a round

Paint over the cooking pots
Take apart the alarm clock
Then we'll mend the sandwiches
With giraffe nails*
So look out!

Now we're gonna go hide
It's your turn to be it
No peeking allowed!
I'm flying away.

CHILDREN'S NURSERY RHYME

---

*The French term *clous de girofle,* which refers to whole cloves, the spice, is often mispronounced by children as *clous de giraffe,* or "giraffe nails." —Trans.

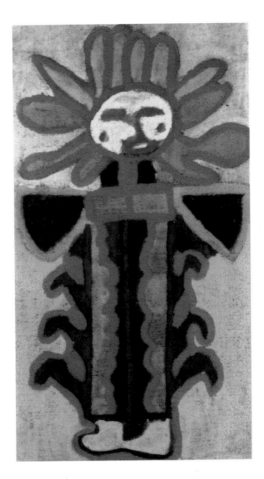

Contents

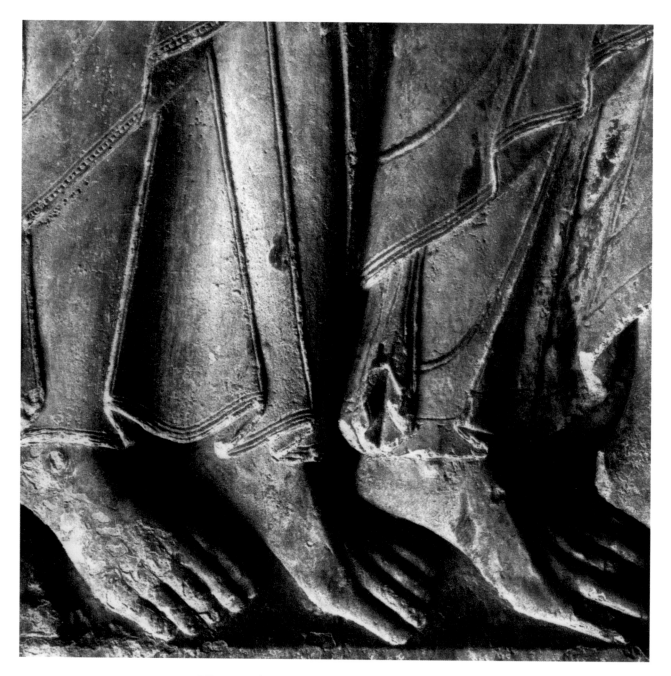

The Apostles, *Silos Abbey. Corner column of the*
Cloister of Silos Abbey, Catalonian Romanesque art

PART ONE

An Introduction to Reflexology

History

The age of reflexology can be calculated in millennia. Over five thousand years ago, the Chinese were practicing pressure-based therapies. The Egyptians knew the art of foot massage, as evidenced by the fresco of a Sixth Dynasty tomb in Saqqarh that shows two men receiving hand and foot treatments.

In the sixteenth century two European doctors published a book devoted to zone therapy. Later, in Leipzig, a Dr. Bell wrote a book on "therapy by pressure," which was practiced during that time in central Europe by people in every level of society, from peasants to courtiers. Various forms of reflexology also existed among indigenous peoples of Africa, Australia, and America.

In 1913, Dr. William Fitzgerald, a general practitioner and ear, nose, and throat specialist in Connecticut, who had earlier worked in hospitals in London, Paris, and Vienna, began research on this technique; it was he who dubbed it "zone therapy." Observing that his operations on the noses and throats of patients were sometimes virtually painless, he deduced intuitively that this local anesthesia was produced by the pressure exercised by the patient on his or her own hand. Over time he gradually integrated this zone therapy into his practice. Eventually he drew from his experience to create a chart on which the body was divided into ten zones (five on either side of a median line), with each zone terminating in a finger and a toe.

The zones apply not just to the body surface but to the insides as well; thus we can speak of dividing the body into ten slices. Fitzgerald and his students found that the longitudinal zones of the feet offered especially effective reflex zones for organs that are in the same body zone. The spine, for example, is located in the first two longitudinal zones of the body's middle line. If you follow these zones inside the legs down to the feet, you will see that these zones run along the inside of the feet. The foot reflex zones for the spine thus lie on the inside edges of the feet. The head zones run across the toes. The shoulder zones run across the ball of the foot in the same way in which the shoulders themselves run across the longitudinal zones of the body. In this way the entire body can be pictured on the feet.

Fitzgerald's reflexology therapy was rapidly refined during the 1930s by another American, Eunice Ingham. Author of the books *Stories the Feet Can Tell* and *Stories the Feet Have Told,* she created plates that showed the corresponding zones for various internal systems on the feet.

While these works constitute the foundation of modern reflexology, they still remained at the empirical stage. Lacking in physiological or anatomical basis, they were too symptomatic and insufficiently scientific in their approach. With the advent of Total Reflexology Therapy, reflexology now has a new scientific path.

The Ten Zones

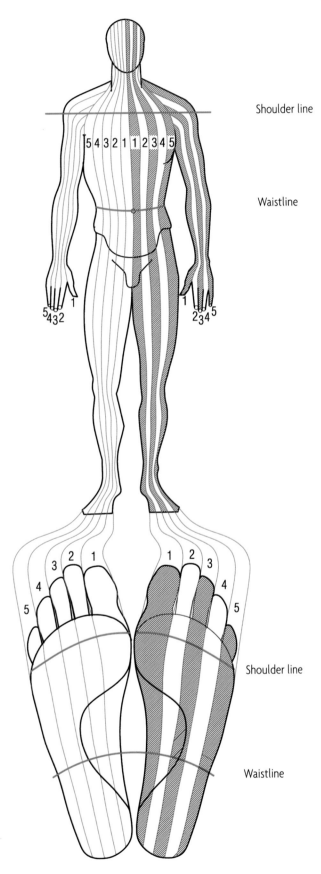

Shoulder line

Waistline

Shoulder line

Waistline

Why Reflexology?

The British neurologist Sir Henry Head (1861–1940) described skin zones, called Head zones, on the human body that correspond to specific internal organs. Illnesses of these organs cause the associated skin zones to "coreact." Reactions can take shape as pain or sensitivity to touch in the respective skin area. Conversely, problems of the organs, especially pain, can be influenced via these areas. Therapeutic treatment can be massages, applications of heat, or injections.

There is a scientific explanation for the relationship between organs and the skin. The skin contains blood vessels and a dense network of nerves. These nerves come as a bundle from the spine. They run not only to the skin but also to the muscles and organs. Thus, in a simplified manner, skin, muscles, and organs are connected with one another via nerves. These connections can be illustrated anatomically and provide an explanation for why organs can be represented as skin zones and why skin zones can influence organs. For example, gallbladder problems can take the form of shoulder or back pain. Pain in the left arm sometimes indicates problems of the heart. Patients with strokes often describe a pain in the left arm.

It is a similar process in the case of foot reflexology. An illness or disturbance in a certain part or area of the body is translated into a painful or especially sensitive zone in the foot. If this zone is then massaged in the proper manner, the symptoms improve or disappear in the respective body part or area.

Practiced on a regular basis, reflexology can lead to a true regeneration of the body. Much like how it carries its own genetic material, the body contains restorative faculties and immunity. Reflexology can stimulate the body's ability to self-heal. Natural medicines work by supporting the body's return to a balanced internal climate: homeostasis, the equilibrium necessary for the harmonious functioning of all the body's systems.

An economical, preventive, and therapeutic method, reflexology affords the practitioner a better grasp of the patient's condition than conventional medicine and a clear understanding of all the pathological conditions that could ensue. It also constitutes an effective supportive therapy for both before and after surgery. Reflexology works best to address disorders affecting normal body function. In serious cases of disease involving cellular degeneration, its effect is only palliative, but it does offer compensation for tissue deterioration.

Reflexology Today

Reflexology is experiencing growing recognition because of its effectiveness in the management of stress and pathological conditions. It is practiced in hospitals and businesses and is reimbursed by some health insurance companies. In Europe, it has greatly reduced absenteeism in the workplace.

Reflexology is less widespread in southern Europe and the United States than in northern Europe despite the growth of training in this practice. Some associations in Europe are currently working to set standards for the teaching of reflexology, but a great effort is still required before the local authorities will accept this discipline as a bona fide medical treatment and encourage its practice by giving grants to students who wish to pursue it.

The Distinctive Features of Total Reflexology Therapy

The holistic principle of the dynamic unity of the body and its self-regulating and self-healing capacities is fundamental to Total Reflexology Therapy. This therapy emphasizes the preponderant role played by the autonomic nervous system, as physical disorders can often be traced back to some dysfunction in this system caused by stress.

In collaboration with my students, I created Total Reflexology Therapy by introducing into reflexology the following:

The Craniosacral System and the Primary Respiratory Mechanism

The craniosacral system is made up of the skull, the spine, the sacrum, and the cerebrospinal fluid (CSF). The bones of the skull move in a rhythm of retraction and expansion (flexing and extending). The primary respiratory mechanism (PRM) can be perceived—at a rhythm of twelve to sixteen pulsations a minute—in all the body's tissues. The CSF, which serves the brain as a kind of shock absorber, relays via the cranial membranes and the spinal cord fluctuations transmitted by the rachidian nerves and the autonomic nervous system. These fluctuations are spread to all the body's cells by means of the fascia. Treating the craniosacral system with reflexology allows the therapist to strengthen the interconnections among connective tissue, bones, muscles, body structures, fluids, and the brain.

Balance of the Sympathetic and Parasympathetic Nervous Systems

The autonomic nervous system is formed by two antagonistic and complementary systems called the sympathetic and parasympathetic. They control the involuntary actions of the body, such as breathing, digestion, elimination, and reproduction. Reflexology treatments can help to keep these parts of the nervous system in balance, contributing to the self-defense, self-balancing, and self-restoring capacities of the body, thus supporting adaptation and protecting life itself.

Stress Syndrome

Through its abilities to adapt to shifting environmental factors, the autonomic nervous system plays an essential role in the reestablishment of balances that have been disrupted by stress. Depending on which "phase of stress" is indicated by the patient's feet, the reflexologist will know, for example, whether to focus the treatment on stimulating the sympathetic or parasympathetic nervous system.

The Occipital Zones

These zones on the skull confirm which zones on the feet need to be worked on, as they provide an exact reflection of the structural, sympathetic, or parasympathetic regions afflicted. The treatment of the affected occipital zone will create a general sense of relaxation to precede any therapeutic reflexology protocol.

Hering's Law

Hering's law provides the basis for meticulously following the evolution or involution of an illness: Symptoms evolve from the outside toward the inside as the illness worsens, then from the inside toward the outside as the patient gets better. Also, the resurgence of symptoms from a past illness heralds improvement. This law enables the therapist to monitor the effects of a treatment, to offer the patient the best possible advice, and to potentially direct him or her to complementary modalities.

Basics of Reflexology

Foot reflexology directly treats the functional illnesses of out-of-balance organs. Any illness should manifest on the foot in the reflex zone of the organ involved; it will betray its presence by a painful sensitivity created by crystalline deposits that congest in the tissues. These sensitive points are also known as the reflex points.

Treatment of these points takes effect by means of the musculo-cutaneous-visceral reflex. Pressure applied to the reflex point creates an electromagnetic wave that follows nerve pathways to reach the spinal cord and then the hypothalamus, which regulates the autonomic nervous system. The hypothalamus processes the information received and induces physiological reactions throughout the body that restore the balance of the autonomic nervous system.

Reflexology acts both gently and deeply. In accordance with naturopathic principles, it restores cellular equilibrium by improving the quality of intracellular and extracellular fluids; circulation of the blood, lymph, and cerebrospinal fluid; and nervous and electromagnetic nutrition by restoring movement of body fluids.

All of this contributes toward positive change in the nervous, hormonal, and lymphatic systems. Reflexology also stimulates the process of elimination, which cleanses the body and thus improves its natural self-healing function. The healing of the cells and tissues on all these levels leads to the restoration of physical, emotional, and mental well-being.

A good foot reflexology massage relaxes and calms the recipient. Aside from good technique, many factors need to be considered for the success of the massage treatment. Here are a few helpful points.

An appealing ambience is important for a good treatment. This means that the massage should take place in a well-ventilated room with a pleasant temperature and that the recipient should be in a comfortable position. The recipient's feet, calves, and, if possible, legs should be free of clothing. If the recipient's pant legs are simply pushed up, make sure that they are not tight, or else they will restrict circulation below the knees, reducing the flow of energy. The massager's clothing should be comfortable and not restrictive.

For the massager, comfortable body position is important. Consider that a full foot reflexology massage will take 30 to 45 minutes. If you become tense during this time because of your own body position, you will have little fun giving foot reflexology massages.

The massage is usually done with the thumbs and tips of the fingers. Make sure that your fingernails do not extend beyond your fingertips, since the massage can otherwise become an unpleasant experience for your partner. Do not give massages with cold hands. The recipient is likely to experience cold hands as being unpleasant. This leads to tension, which in turn nullifies any beneficial effect of the massage.

The recipient's feet must be warm and dry. Cold feet are the most common reason for the failure of a foot massage. If the recipient's feet are cold, warm them either with a heat lamp, a warm footbath, or with a hot water bottle wrapped in a towel.

Massage gently. Begin the massage with a few introductory strokes over the whole area before you begin addressing the individual zones.

Keep eye contact with your partner. By looking at your partner, you will know immediately how your massage is being received. Ask your partner about his or her sensations. It is important that you communicate during the massage and give your partner the opportunity to ask questions. However, do not make diagnoses or suppositions about illnesses if certain zones are sensitive.

Sole of Foot

Top of Foot

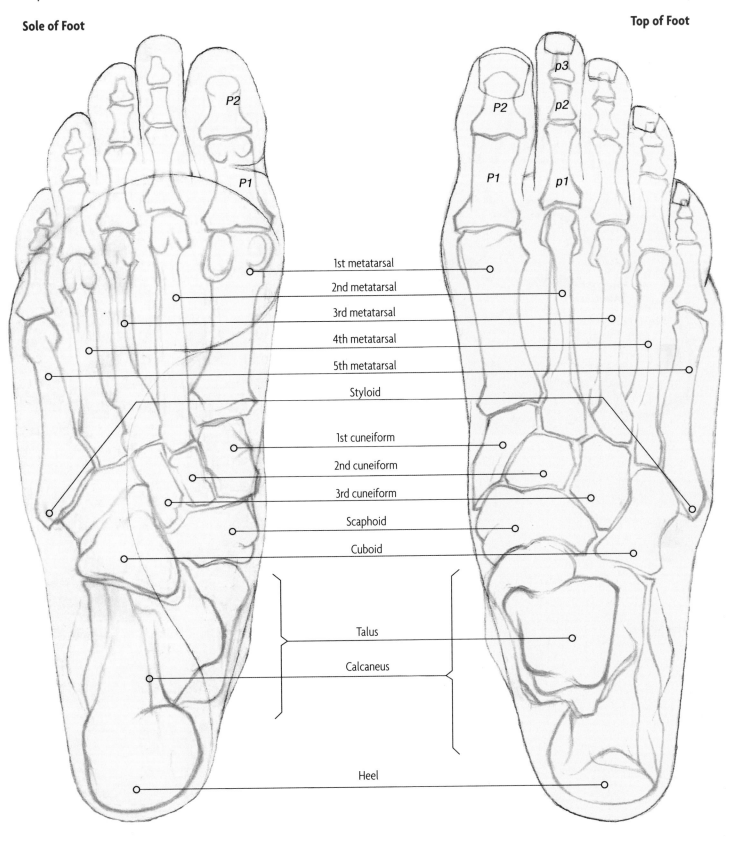

P2

P1

p3

P2

p2

P1

p1

1st metatarsal

2nd metatarsal

3rd metatarsal

4th metatarsal

5th metatarsal

Styloid

1st cuneiform

2nd cuneiform

3rd cuneiform

Scaphoid

Cuboid

Talus

Calcaneus

Heel

The Bones of the Foot

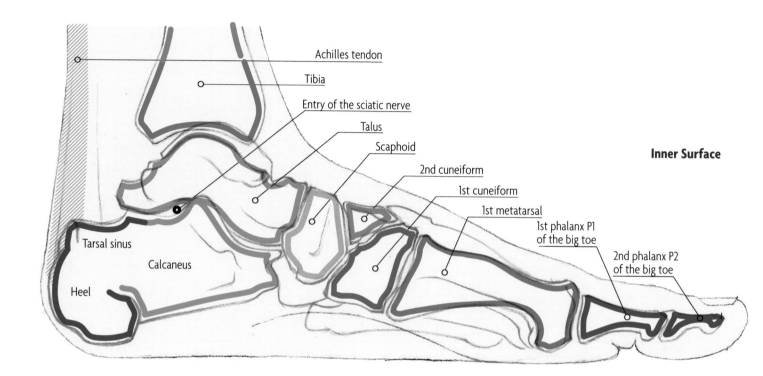

Achilles tendon
Tibia
Entry of the sciatic nerve
Talus
Scaphoid
2nd cuneiform
1st cuneiform
1st metatarsal
1st phalanx P1 of the big toe
2nd phalanx P2 of the big toe

Inner Surface

Tarsal sinus
Calcaneus
Heel

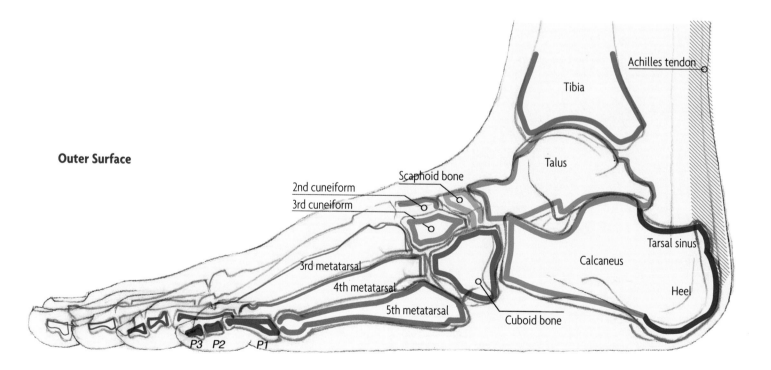

Outer Surface

Achilles tendon
Tibia
Talus
Tarsal sinus
Calcaneus
Heel
Scaphoid bone
2nd cuneiform
3rd cuneiform
3rd metatarsal
4th metatarsal
5th metatarsal
Cuboid bone
P3   P2   P1

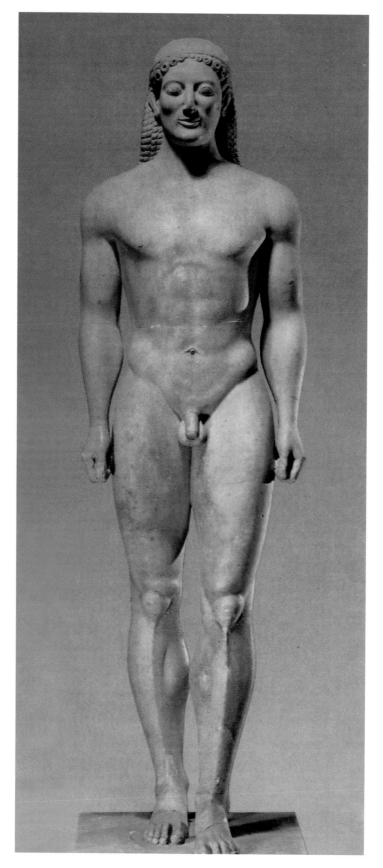

Kouros, 525 BCE, National Archaeological Museum of Athens

PART TWO

The Therapeutic Experience

Total Reflexology Treatment

The foot is a reflection of the human being in its entirety: not only physical, emotional, and mental, but temporal as well. It carries the stigmas of the individual's past and the promises of his or her future. This is something the reflexologist should always bear in mind when consulting with a patient.

Indications

Reflexology can successfully restore the circulatory, nervous, immune, digestive, hormonal, and structural systems to normal functioning. It is equally valuable as a preliminary treatment before osteopathic and chiropractic manipulations, and as an adjunct therapy before and after operations. Reflexology is now authorized and even recommended by professors in the field of medicine.

If homeostasis is no longer possible, Total Reflexology Therapy does bring comfort to patients with serious illnesses and helps them tolerate their medications.

Before beginning any work on a patient, the practitioner should first observe some basic details.

The Patient's Gait

Does the patient walk with a spring in his step? This reveals the harmonious development of the ligaments and muscles. With flexibility and agility? This is a good indication of the absence of tension. Is the gait rigid? This reveals either some physical disorder—muscular, arthritic, or neurological—or a rigid mental attitude. Does the patient hammer the ground with her heels? This signals a strong will and the desire to assert one's territorial boundaries.

Posture

The position of the head is quite important. It should be held straight and slightly raised, with the shoulders relaxed and open—all indications of a relaxed state.

When the body leans forward, it creates pressure in the cervical region and on the frontal portion of the brain, as well as on the lumbar spine, because the body's weight is poorly distributed. This may reveal an impulsive character with a tendency to rush ahead; anxiety and a general lack of ease result. This posture may also cause pressure on the rib cage and the abdominal organs. Respiratory capacity is then reduced, and blood circulates poorly, no longer reaching all parts of the body. Among the health disorders associated with hunched shoulders and poor posture are asthma, bronchitis, and other respiratory problems.

Seated Posture

Is the patient relaxed? Do her hands and legs fall naturally into place? If they are crossed or fidgety, this reveals a lack of ease.

Oral Expression

Does the patient express himself in a well-modulated and harmonious tone of voice? Or is his voice sharp and his delivery abrupt?

Skin Tone

Is the skin of the patient pale, pink, gray, yellow, red, or brown? Skin coloration can indicate certain deficiencies in the body. Is the patient suffering from acne or rough patches on her skin?

The Clinical Aspect of the Foot

Observe the color and form. Note the imperfections and watch for corns, warts, scars, and damaged toenails. The foot's temperature reveals the state of the circulatory system. Athlete's foot indicates an unbalanced pH of the foot's secretions. Viral warts indicate a nutritional deficiency.

Damp skin indicates strong emotions and disturbance in the autonomic nervous system. Hyperkeratosis, or a thickening of the outer layer of the skin on the foot, reveals the elimination of toxins. It's best to clear away this protective layer before beginning reflexology treatments.

It is sometimes necessary to consult a podiatrist before beginning therapeutic treatment.

Listening to the Patient

The practitioner must be a good listener. This is of fundamental importance. His or her listening must be active and attentive. Responses to the patient's questions should be spontaneous and given in a calm voice. The practitioner should listen without judging, interrupting, or changing the subject. It's best not to rush the patient or take her out of her natural rhythm. Trust is a very important factor in the healing process.

The practitioner should take notes on the patient's previous history, illnesses, surgeries, and all past and current medical treatments.

Beginning to Work

Touch

Touching is a means of gaining entrance into the psyche. It leads the patient to better self-awareness. All touch is an exchange and an act of sharing. The reflexologist's touch should be gentle, calm, precise, and attentive.

Occipital Palpation

Before beginning the actual treatment of the foot, the practitioner should treat the occipital zones. These will reveal the disorders that will be found on the foot during the course of the therapy. (For more, see the chapter The Occipital Zones and the Ten Reflex Zones.)

Technique

Once the patient is comfortably seated or lying down, the therapist (who should also be comfortable) should go over both feet with his or her hands in order to determine skin quality and temperature. This will also relax the feet and loosen the joints.

The practitioner should listen quite carefully, at the levels of head and foot, to the quality of the movement of the cerebrospinal fluid (CSF). The massage should be performed by pressing the thumb on the zone to be treated, moving it in a circular motion, without disengaging from the skin. This pattern mimics the helicoidal movement of the DNA.

The actual massage of individual zones is done using different pressure techniques that use the fingertips, especially the tips of the thumb and index finger. Pressure can be applied in two ways: a steady pressure, or one that moves through a zone point by point.

The Thumb or Caterpillar Walk

The thumb or caterpillar walk is one of the most commonly used moves in foot reflexology. Pressure is applied vertically on the tissue, and the following release and small movement of the thumb onto the next point is reminiscent of the walk of a caterpillar.

While you are exerting pressure with your thumb, a counterbalance is needed, which is provided by the fingers. From the side, your hand looks like it is curving or forming a U shape around the foot.

The Technique of Steady Pressure

For painful or especially sensitive zones you can use steady pressure with the thumb. The movement of the caterpillar is skipped, and instead pressure is applied exactly to the sensitive or painful spot and kept steady for a longer period of time. Again, place your thumb flat on the targeted area, bend your thumb, and in this position apply a steady pressure.

The duration of the pressure can be from 1 to 2 minutes. Here, too, the previous rule applies: the intensity and duration of the pressure depend on the needs of your patient. Steady pressure will often resolve the painful zones. But definitely respect the pain limits of your patient. If the sensitivity of the zone does not decrease, you can massage the zone again in a later pass.

The Caterpillar Walk with the Index Finger

You can massage by "walking" with your index finger just as you can with your thumb. This variation of the caterpillar walk is especially good for zones that because of their sensitivity do not respond well to strong pressure. It is used primarily on the top of the foot, since there are bones and tendons directly under the skin in this area. As with the thumb walk, the caterpillar walk with the index finger can be split up into several phases. In the first phase, you place the index finger flat on the skin without applying any pressure. In the second phase, you bend the finger in its middle joint and, as you bend it, start applying pressure to the tissue. Here, the thumb is the counterbalance. In the final phase, you release the pressure and roll the tip of the finger until it come to a rest flat against the skin, again not applying any pressure. From this position you can begin the next pressure movement. As with the thumb walk, with the index-finger walk you work point by point through the selected zone.

The Tweezers Move

In the tweezers move you work with the tips of the thumb and the index finger. With this move you will reach the "swimming skins" or membranes between the toes. Take the skin between the flat parts of your thumb and index finger and slightly pull the skin out in the direction of the toes. This helps the circulation in these zones. The pull as well as the pressure applied is steady. Switch between pull and relaxation in rhythm with the breathing of your patient.

With the tweezers grip you can also massage the individual toes point by point. Beginning at the base of the toe, apply pressure for a moment, then release it. Work point by point from the base of the toes to the tips.

If a reflex point proves painful to the touch, lightly massage all over the foot with essential oils to prepare the patient for treatment. Wipe away the excess in order to keep your fingers from slipping.

The intensity of the pressure applied and the duration and frequency of the sessions will all vary according to the age of the patient, his or her tolerance to pain, the tone of the skin and of the underlying tissue, and the patient's state of health and degree of vital energy. For children, the sessions should be briefer but scheduled close together. For the elderly, the sessions should also be brief but should be scheduled more infrequently.

The End of the Session

Once the treatment session has ended, the reflexologist should again listen to the CSF. Have the patient take several deep and conscious breaths and relax for a few minutes.

Each session should last about an hour. At the treatment's end, the patient will first demonstrate a sense of cold. She may shiver, yawn, and stretch.

Effects will be noted on the liver, gallbladder, kidneys, skin, and so forth: these are eliminatory reactions. The patient will get better in his own time, depending on his nature, his capacity to be open and receptive, and the chronicity of his condition.

Contraindications

There are no specific contraindications to reflexology treatment. However, it is wise to be cautious with cases involving degenerative diseases or serious diseases with an immunodepressant component, such as cancer and AIDS; viral and bacterial pneumonia or serious bronchial obstructions; or anything that contributes to the deterioration of the physical body, such as internal and cerebral hemorrhaging. In the case of pregnancy, it is better to avoid applying treatment to certain zones of the foot and to respect the lunar calendar.

It is always possible to bring relief to pain, stress, and fear, however. Total Reflexology Therapy permits patients to better tolerate functional disorders and pain caused both by illnesses of organic origin and by the medications customarily prescribed for serious diseases.

The Therapeutic Experience of Reflexology

In order to be healthy, it's important to cultivate a healthy lifestyle, with good nutrition and regular physical exercise. Reflexology can be as effective as acupuncture, homeopathy, phytotherapy, and psychotherapy at keeping health in balance.

When a patient seeks help for excess weight, sleeplessness, poor digestion, painful menstrual periods, or infertility, the first step taken by the practitioner should always be to assess the extent of the patient's stress, the extent of the disorder, as well as how much degeneration has taken place in the tissues.

Reflexology can be just as easily applied to a newborn as to someone in the twilight of life. For birth-induced cranial compression, which can manifest as crying day and night, regurgitation of milk, eczema, constipation, or diarrhea, craniosacral therapy applied to the feet will be able to provide the necessary relief.

It should be noted that a difficult birth can traumatize the craniosacral system, throwing the posture out of alignment and causing pain. If this condition goes without treatment, it can become permanent. Arthrosis of the vertebral column, at whatever level of the spine it occurs, can be successfully treated with reflexology.

In the elderly, rigidity in the joints can cause considerable pain along the spinal column. An elderly person suffering from exhaustion, insomnia, or depression or exhibiting any chronic symptoms will feel better and recover energy following a general reflexology treatment.

Example of a Treatment Plan: Obesity

The origin of excess poundage is varied and can be due to anxiety, stress, or medications (birth control pills, antibiotics, stimulants, relaxants, multiple vaccinations). These extra pounds often yield to regular reflexology treatments accompanied by a balanced diet, relaxation, and physical exercise.

This condition is improved by treatment of the hormonal glands, particularly the thyroid, adrenal, pituitary, and pineal glands. Disorders of the thyroid can often cause fatigue, depression, weight gain, and a general lack of well-being both mentally and emotionally. Dysfunctions of the adrenal glands inhibit the ability to adapt to stress and can make rest nearly impossible, bringing the patient to total exhaustion.

Obesity can also result from an imbalanced autonomic nervous system. An overactive sympathetic nervous system will show up as too much energy; an overactive parasympathetic system will appear as a lack of energy. The exhaustion of both these systems leads to sleep disorders.

Through study of the recurring symptoms over the course of treatment, the practitioner will carefully analyze the disorders of each individual patient. All excess weight involves an energetic imbalance that inhibits the body from burning off excess fats. This will then affect the sympathetic nervous system, resulting in slower liver, spleen, pancreatic, and intestinal function. Excess fats will then build up in the tissues of the body.

If the body is functioning as if in slow motion and proves to be thoroughly clogged, if it turns out to be storing toxins in its tissues, then the reflexology treatment will be applied to the lymph and vein network systems as well as to the digestive, hormonal, and nervous systems, especially the autonomic nervous system.

For a patient suffering from a high degree of anxiety, the zones calling out for treatment will be the abdomen, the solar plexus, the stomach, and the intestines. If the traumas are far in the past, then treatment should also cover the zone corresponding to the kidneys and adrenal glands in order to regulate the compulsions of the stomach.

The practitioner should analyze the patient's emotional states and psychological coping mechanisms, along with their consequences on physical well-being. The loss of weight will be effective only after all the shocks and traumas—emotional and physical—that were its cause have been thoroughly erased from cellular memory. For example, repressed and forgotten emotions—an absence of love, perhaps—are often compensated for with extra food. Everything that does not find expression is stored away in cellular memory and in the body's tissues, where it disrupts the well-being of the individual, who will be out of balance in both her inner world and her body. The body also seeks compensations, in ways that are too often self-destructive. The patient who wishes to lose weight must be willing to sort things out emotionally.

Reflexology helps to deprogram the mechanisms and habits that have been rooted in the body since childhood. Part of the practitioner's job is to help the patient locate why and how past traumas buried away in memory have created his or her particular physical disorders and to show the patient why it's crucial to reprogram the harmful habits that have been in place for so long.

This reprogramming also has two components:

1. The psychological data from the past—the events that brought about the disorders being treated—must be brought to light. (The patient must express himself.) The past events must be reframed and resolved in positive terms.
2. The patient must adopt a healthier lifestyle in order to enjoy better physical health. This means that she should breathe in a way that reoxygenates the body; she should build new eating habits; and she should exercise on a regular basis.

The general treatment should be followed by a craniosacral treatment.

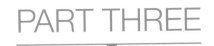

PART THREE

Overview of Human Anatomy and Physiology

The Cell

The cell is the functional unit of the organs and systems to which it belongs. Bearing its own characteristic DNA, each cell is a complex universe made up of multiple energetic fields that are both interconnected and interdependent, with levels of precisely harmonized organization.

Each cell is the seat of chemical reactions and is self-replicating. Each leads its own life and plays a role in the overall functioning of the body. The cells are immersed in an extracellular fluid whose state must remain stable for their survival. The stability of the nutrients and minerals that create this fluid depends upon the membranes of the cells and the osmotic process between two membranes (intracellular and extracellular). It is the role of a cellular membrane, by means of an electrochemical gradient and a selective permeability, to regulate the passage of the substances entering and exiting the cell.

The cell is a miniature factory. The products of its labor are employed toward its continued survival; some parts are stored, such as fats, and some sent away, such as the waste products created by the cell's activity. One could say that the functioning of the organs depends upon the functioning of the individual cells, which in turn depends upon the constant maintenance of a harmonious inner environment. Both cells and organs have a role to play in this internal maintenance process of homeostasis.

DNA-RNA

The study of the mechanics of DNA (deoxyribonucleic acid) explains the formidable healing powers inherent to life. The body possesses its own internal doctor; human beings and their cells intuitively know how to heal themselves. This explains how humans have managed to survive over the course of millions of years of evolution.

In all organisms DNA takes the same form: a very large molecule in the shape of a double helix with two chains of nucleotides woven around each other and interconnected. These DNA nucleotides, which take four different forms, are the "letters" of the genetic code of information that is essential for the construction and function of life.

DNA reproduces by duplication, each time transmitting its genetic information from one cell to another and from one generation to another. It transcribes this information in another macromolecule, RNA (ribonucleic acid), which travels from the cell's nucleus and translates the genetic information as required for the manufacture of proteins specific to the structure and function of each particular organism. Reproduction, transcription, and translation are clearly the vital mechanisms of life. After DNA delivers its coded messages to its active twin, RNA, through "locks," RNA then enters the cell and distributes parcels of information to thousands of enzymes.

Enzymes are proteins endowed with highly elevated catalytic power. They accelerate vital reactions in order to maintain the vital functions. Their three-dimensional configuration allows them to bind easily with other molecules, hastening their reaction and transformation.

Polymerase I directs the replication of DNA and also plays an essential role in the repair of gaps in the DNA. The reparative system of the cell is always vigilant and in constant action. It eliminates damaged structures and replaces them with healthy ones. It ceaselessly monitors the maintenance of normal structure and

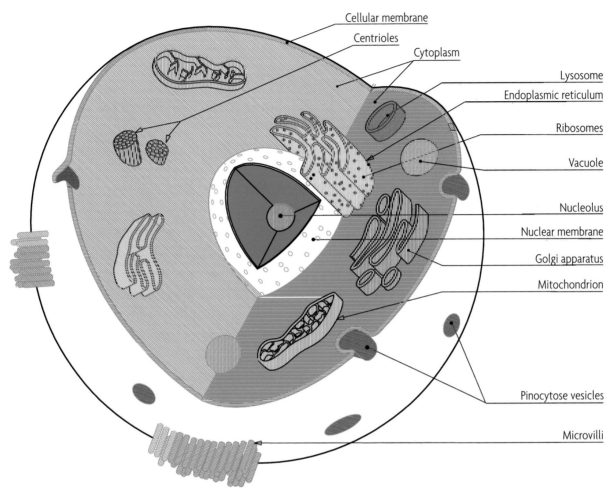

Cellular membrane
Centrioles
Cytoplasm
Lysosome
Endoplasmic reticulum
Ribosomes
Vacuole
Nucleolus
Nuclear membrane
Golgi apparatus
Mitochondrion
Pinocytose vesicles
Microvilli

function. The appearance of a lesion or error automatically stimulates the reparative process; therefore, the healing is spontaneous—the body heals itself.

At every stage there is an exchange of energy and information. Thus, metabolism is more than just a simple act of combustion; it is an intelligent action stored in the DNA and transmitted through coded information for each cell function.

Each strand of DNA contains within itself the code for the entire human being, with all its organs, biological rhythms, humors, and cycles of development. Coiled around itself, it contains twenty-two pairs of chromosomes, plus one more single chromosome for the differentiation of the sexes (XX woman; XY man). A human being develops from a single embryonic cell containing its complete program in its DNA.

The Effect of Metals upon the Cells

Metals represent the memory of the solar system within us, materializing in some way the bond between Earth and the other planets. These "alchemical" metals (gold, silver, mercury, copper, iron, tin, and lead) carry out transmutations in a cell; they also activate the cell's biological mechanisms and its sequencing of memory.

The metalloids (calcium, magnesium, sodium, potassium, and iodine) play a structuring role. They strengthen the cohesiveness of the DNA and of the nucleus. By attaching themselves to the outside of the double helix, they increase the stability of the form. Other metals (silver, mercury) bond to the interior of the double helix, on the base pairs, and induce instability and change. These other metals are specifically implicated in sites of mutation. The role these metals play is crucial to the process of evolution and to the management of the crises that bring about this evolution. Depending on the case, either they open the form, bringing about a crisis of transformation, or they provide it with the strength it needs to resist external pressure.

Etienne Guille, of the Orsay School, has observed that certain sites of chromosomes are particularly rich in metals. Through constant movements, these metals lodge themselves in specific sites of DNA reception around the nucleus of the cell. Each metal vibrates according to specific directions coded within the cell. This vibratory energy is a factor in the evolution of form.

Vibrational fields connect the human being to all forms of life through both time and space. What an individual experiences is imprinted upon these fields and memorized in the very nuclei of his or her cells. Therefore, there's a collective influence, through resonance, on all individuals sharing the same fields of consciousness or energy. This, in a nutshell, is how information is distributed holographically. The fields of energy that run through the body resonate and interact in much the same way that information is transmitted holographically. Quantum theory and Kirlian photographs demonstrate that the human being is not so much a dense, physical entity as a luminous, sonorous, and colorful energetic being.

A cell that becomes physically isolated shuts down its capacity to receive information through its membranes and no longer communicates with the cells that feed and sustain it. It dries up in a state of sclerosis, then either dies or turns anarchically against the body. This cellular isolation, triggered by the body's reaction to suffering, then brings about an overall reduction in the potential for vital existence. In a study involving more than fifteen thousand individuals, Dr. Ryke Geerd Hamer demonstrated that malignant tumors always correlated with a dramatic event that had never been verbalized and was most often experienced in isolation. Of course nutrition, pollution, and viruses can be held equally responsible, but the emotional state still plays the dominant role because it affects brain functioning, and it is the brain that organizes the body in function and form, thus maintaining its overall health. When the immune system has been weakened by a tragic experience, identifying the trauma and bringing the buried emotions into awareness can inhibit the spread of disease.

The reflexologist should always bear in mind that the pathology is only the visible part of the iceberg, the consequence and not the cause of an imbalance. The body is the bearer of millions of years of wisdom, woven into each cell. We must know how to listen to it. Our vital force is consciousness; consciousness is life itself.

DNA

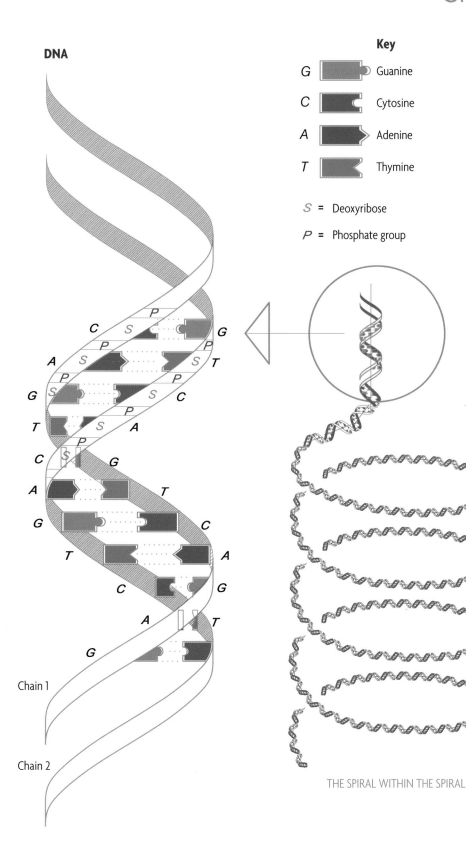

Key

G		Guanine
C		Cytosine
A		Adenine
T		Thymine

S = Deoxyribose

P = Phosphate group

Chain 1

Chain 2

THE SPIRAL WITHIN THE SPIRAL

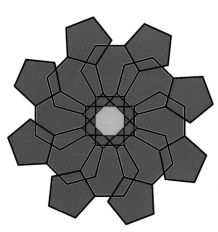

Mandala obtained by projecting a DNA molecule on a plane perpendicular to the axis of the double helix

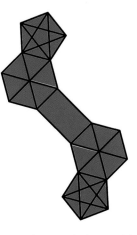

Schematic depiction of the hexagonal and pentagonal components of the DNA spiral

The Embryological Basis
of Reflexology

Looking at embryos and how they develop (embryology) makes it possible to understand how a zone on the skin can have a relationship with a particular organ, bone, muscle, fascia, or the nervous or lymphatic system.

The three embryonic germ layers—ectoderm, mesoderm, and endoderm—develop out of the amniotic cavity, initiating the conduction of the mono- and polysynaptic reflexes. The ectoderm (the outermost layer of the embryo) is the source of brain and skin. The mesoderm (the middle layer) is the source of skeleton, soft tissue, and muscles. The endoderm (the innermost layer) is the source of the digestive system (from mouth to anus).

The development of the embryo from the three germ layers takes place in the following sequence:

Phase 1: Three layers of differentiated cells form the embryonic disk within the amniotic cavity. The neural fold and fissure appear in the groove of the ectoderm.

Phase 2: The neural folds grow larger, topped by the neural crest.

Phases 3 and 4: The neural folds fuse to form the neural tube. The mesoderm differentiates to produce bony, muscular, and connective tissue. The crescent formed by the endoderm closes into a tube.

Phase 5: Skin, the digestive tube, the neural tube, and the intestines are all now separate entities. The neural crest cells develop into the dorsal root ganglia.

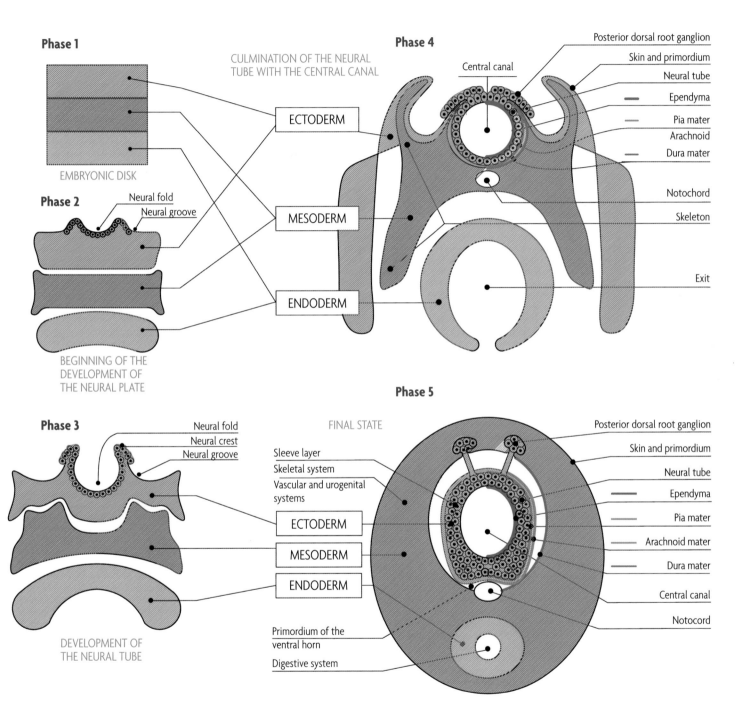

Phase 1

EMBRYONIC DISK

Phase 2

Neural fold
Neural groove

BEGINNING OF THE
DEVELOPMENT OF
THE NEURAL PLATE

Phase 3

Neural fold
Neural crest
Neural groove

ECTODERM
MESODERM
ENDODERM

DEVELOPMENT OF
THE NEURAL TUBE

CULMINATION OF THE NEURAL
TUBE WITH THE CENTRAL CANAL

ECTODERM

MESODERM

ENDODERM

Phase 4

Central canal

Posterior dorsal root ganglion
Skin and primordium
Neural tube
Ependyma
Pia mater
Arachnoid
Dura mater

Notochord

Skeleton

Exit

Phase 5

FINAL STATE

Sleeve layer
Skeletal system
Vascular and urogenital
systems

ECTODERM
MESODERM
ENDODERM

Primordium of the
ventral horn

Digestive system

Posterior dorsal root ganglion
Skin and primordium
Neural tube
Ependyma
Pia mater
Arachnoid mater
Dura mater
Central canal
Notocord

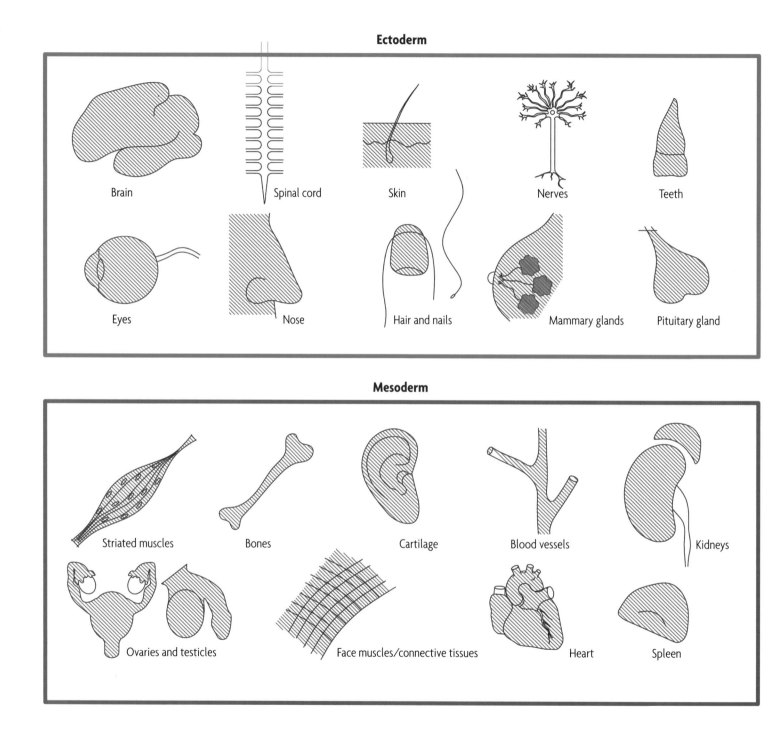

Ectoderm

Brain

Spinal cord

Skin

Nerves

Teeth

Eyes

Nose

Hair and nails

Mammary glands

Pituitary gland

Mesoderm

Striated muscles

Bones

Cartilage

Blood vessels

Kidneys

Ovaries and testicles

Face muscles/connective tissues

Heart

Spleen

Endoderm

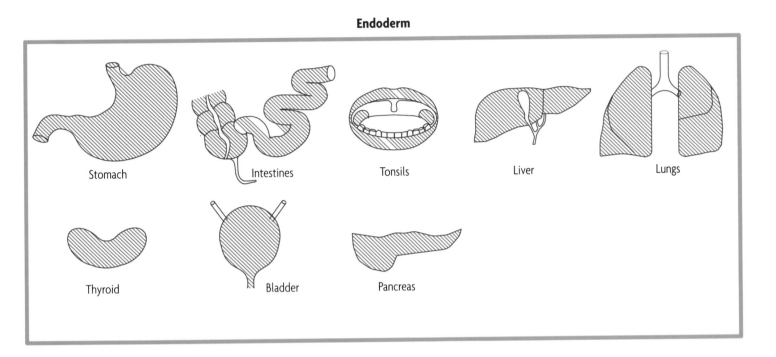

Stomach   Intestines   Tonsils   Liver   Lungs

Thyroid   Bladder   Pancreas

The Reflex Arc

Stimulation of the skin calls forth a response in a specific zone—articular, visceral, muscular, and so on—through a mono- or polysynaptic reflex arc. The reverse is equally true: the nerve impulse exiting the medulla reaches the surface area, carrying up information harvested from the depths, and reveals the zones that are sensitive or painful to signal old and new disorders of varying degrees of seriousness.

This round-trip journey of information is called biofeedback. It is a retroactive system that ensures the supervision and regulation of the entire body.

A specific zone on the skin will "metamerically" reflect its organ counterpart.

The Reflex Arc
Monosynaptic Reflex Arc

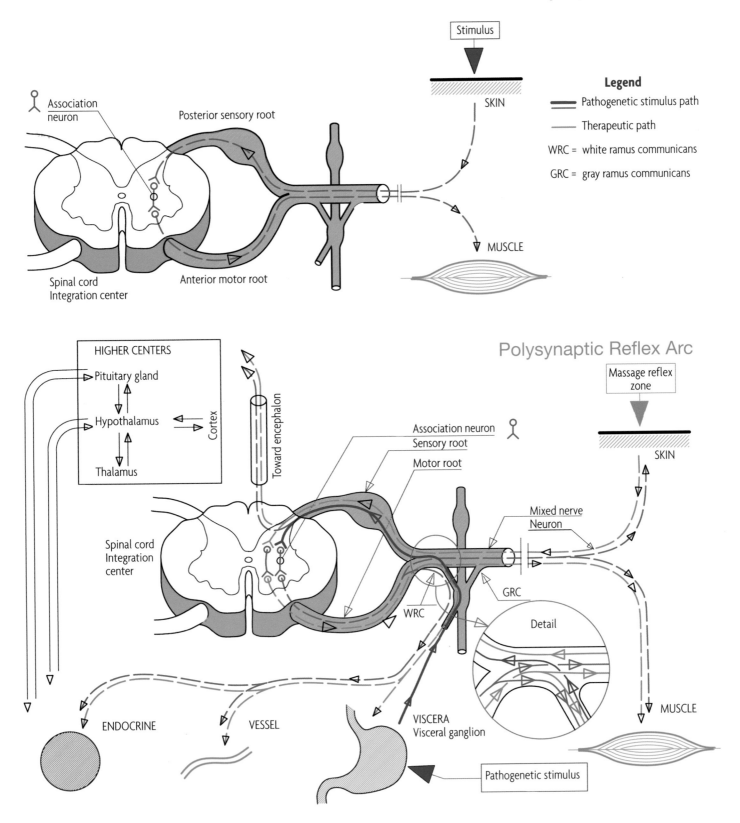

Polysynaptic Reflex Arc

Legend

— Pathogenetic stimulus path
— Therapeutic path

WRC = white ramus communicans
GRC = gray ramus communicans

Stimulus

SKIN

MUSCLE

Association neuron

Posterior sensory root

Spinal cord
Integration center

Anterior motor root

HIGHER CENTERS

Pituitary gland

Hypothalamus

Cortex

Thalamus

Toward encephalon

Spinal cord
Integration center

Association neuron
Sensory root

Motor root

Mixed nerve
Neuron

Massage reflex zone

SKIN

GRC

WRC

Detail

ENDOCRINE

VESSEL

VISCERA
Visceral ganglion

Pathogenetic stimulus

MUSCLE

Biotypes or Somatotypes

As we have seen earlier, the body is the result of the organization of the three original embryonic germ layers, or tissues; for this reason, a predominance of one of these tissues over the others is possible in each individual. The preponderant tissue is then responsible for certain tendencies in the autonomic nervous system of the individual. These sympathetic or parasympathetic tendencies could be misunderstood as signs of pathology in the autonomic nervous system; there is no basis for this, however, as these states are purely physiological.

This brings us to the notion of the human biotype. Particular characteristics—embryonic, morphological, autonomic, metabolic, and temperamental—are specific to each type.

The evaluation of a patient's biotype and attendant pathological tendencies is an essential prerequisite to the reflexology treatment. The biotype guides the therapist in determining the length, intensity, and frequency of treatment sessions and also in advising the patient on matters of nutrition and healthy living.

The Different Biotypes

Each of the three biotypes has its corresponding autonomic nervous system and its own emotional makeup. However, biotypes are rarely pure, and most people exhibit a blending of traits. For example, someone might be thin in the upper body and more rounded below the waist.

The Ectomorph

The ectomorph is thin and lacks definition in the curve of his spinal column. His bones are long and his muscles undeveloped. This delicate individual has a long neck, a narrow chest, and his lower limbs are long but weak. He tends to be stiff.

Anxious, hypersensitive, and hypernervous, this individual is an intellectual, often with ambition. Tense and cerebral, he functions by force of will, his mannerisms often strained. He worries much more about his own health and well-being than about those of others. He craves solitude.

The ectomorph is catabolic and rapidly uses up his energy. A "functional" type (see the next section, entitled "Morphology and the Stress Syndrome"), he is

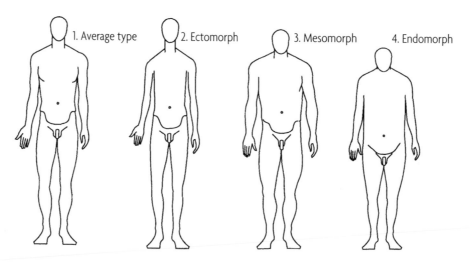

1. Average type   2. Ectomorph   3. Mesomorph   4. Endomorph

always complaining of something (spasms, muscle tension, high blood pressure).

He has a poor appetite and suffers from bad digestion, as his stomach is of a longer and thinner shape than normal. Reflexology sessions should be short so as to avoid overstimulation. Craniosacral treatment is indicated for this biotype.

The Mesomorph

The mesomorph is an athlete; he is of the "structural" type. This individual's athletic build is characterized by large, muscular shoulders and massive limbs. His skin is thick. The mesomorph tends toward high blood pressure. He is hardy, adapts well to his surroundings, and is self-willed, dynamic, and determined rather than ambitious.

Through overexertion and overeating, the mesomorph can destroy his body and is subject to serious diseases such as arteriosclerosis, fibrosis, heart disease, and cerebral thrombosis. Because of his "structural" type, the mesomorph is predisposed to sclerosis, osteoarthritis, and kidney stones.

The body's structural elements and muscle, ligament, and bone tissue constitute this individual's most vulnerable areas. In reflexology, general treatments are highly indicated for this biotype.

The Endomorph

The endomorph has a spinal column with pronounced curvature. This individual tends to be small and round, with a large chest and short legs. He shows little muscular development, tends toward fat, and suffers from premature baldness. His skin is soft, with oily tendencies. This individual is quite flexible and relaxed. He is of the "anabolic" type.

The endomorph has a tendency to be driven by his or her parasympathetic nervous system. More often introverted and phlegmatic in appearance, he is peaceful, exhibiting no aggressive behaviors. He likes company, and even needs it.

A heavy eater, he is likely to show evidence of diseases related to excessive bile, such as those affecting the gallbladder and liver. The internal secretions produced by the ectomorph's body are noteworthy.

This individual suffers from diseases of a functional nature. In reflexology, the appropriate treatment consists of balancing the sympathetic and parasympathetic nervous systems, and work on the plexuses is essential.

Structural and Functional Types

Functional types are hyperresponsive and overreact. Structural types are hyporesponsive and underreact. Consequently, structural types may experience some progressive deterioration with no external sign of disease for a long period of time.

For example, dyspnea (difficult breathing) is structural in nature if it occurs during exertion. It classifies as a functional disorder if it takes place when the individual is seated.

The functional type has strong immune resistance. The defense system of the structural type is not as sound. He or she may be sick for weeks on end.

The spinal column is the structure that governs function. It should be balanced and flexible so as not to obstruct the flow of nerve impulses. Any such blockage could bring about an overstimulation to the organs. Conversely, just as an organ can be overstimulated by blockages in the spine, one can stimulate an organ by following the vertebral column on the reflexology zones of the feet (or hands), even if no stiffness or blockage is apparent.

It is important to be cautious in the choice of treatment for different biotypes in order to avoid any boomerang effects. For example, an injury in the thoracic vertebrae (part of the sympatheic nervous system) upsets the sympathetic nervous system for the ectomorph. This type's sympathetic system, already highly active, is easily overstimulated. When this happens, the energetic harmony between the parasympathetic and sympathetic systems is disrupted and minor mental disorders may result.

Similarly, an endomorph may be overly stimulated during the releasing of joints in the sacral or cervical regions of the spine. Because this type is ruled by the parasympathetic system, he or she will then be thrown out of balance.

It can never be repeated too many times that it is necessary first and foremost to treat the person and not the symptom.

The Nervous System

The nervous system consists of the autonomic nervous system, the central nervous system, and the peripheral nervous system.

The Autonomic Nervous System

The autonomic nervous system could also be described as the involuntary nervous system. It consists of two antagonistic yet complementary systems that each balances out the other: the sympathetic nervous system, which plays the role of the accelerator, and the parasympathetic nervous system, which plays the role of the decelerator.

The craniosacral system is divided into sections dominated by either the parasympathetic or the sympathetic system. The cranial and spinal parasympathetic system goes from the foramen magnum (the opening in the skull through which the spinal cord passes) to the seventh cervical vertebra C7 (space C7/T1) and includes the cranial nerves. The superior and inferior cervical ganglia, along with the stellate ganglion, are sympathetic but are located within this parasympathetic region.

The other parasympathetic region is located in the pelvis. It goes from the second lumbar L2 (space L2/L3) to the fourth sacral S4 (space S4/S5) and includes the sacral nerves. Its neurotransmitter is acetylcholine.

The sympathetic region of the spine goes from the first thoracic (T1) to the second lumbar L2 (space L2/L3). Its neurotransmitter is noradrenaline.

The medullary centers of the spinal cord govern elements of both the visceral region and the autonomic functions of the somatic regions, including vascular, glandular, and sudoriparous functions. The visceral centers are located from T1 to L3 in the sympathetic region of the spine, and the somatic centers extend over the full length of the spinal cord.

Each part of the body is innervated by these two systems, which complement each other. At the junction where T12 meets L1, the spinal cord comes to an end, but the fibers that are inherent to both systems continue to extend farther and innervate the more distant zones.

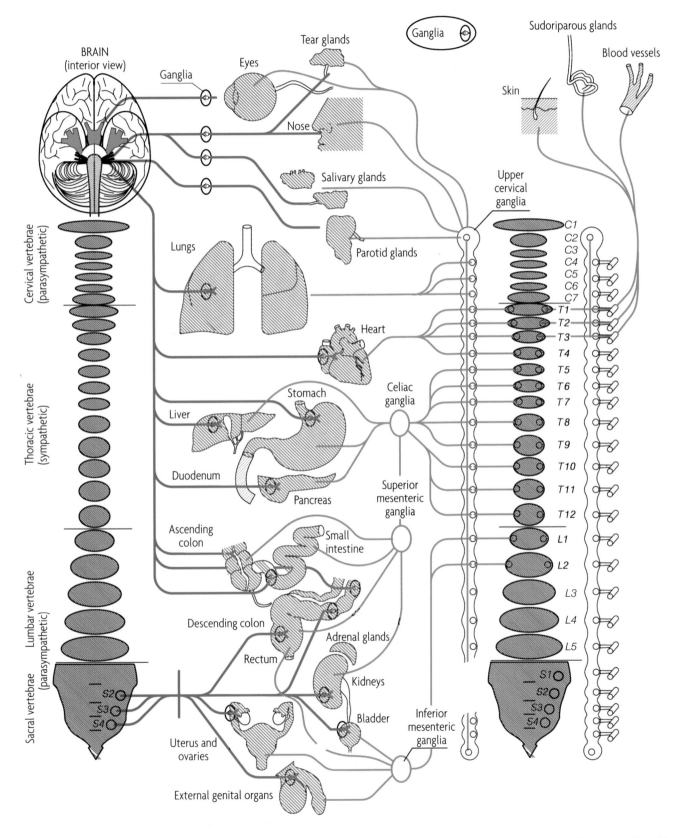

Ganglia

Sudoriparous glands

Blood vessels

Skin

BRAIN
(interior view)

Ganglia

Eyes

Tear glands

Nose

Salivary glands

Parotid glands

Upper
cervical
ganglia

Lungs

Heart

Stomach

Liver

Celiac
ganglia

Duodenum

Pancreas

Ascending
colon

Small
intestine

Superior
mesenteric
ganglia

Descending colon

Adrenal glands

Rectum

Kidneys

Bladder

Inferior
mesenteric
ganglia

Uterus and
ovaries

External genital organs

Cervical vertebrae
(parasympathetic)

Thoracic vertebrae
(sympathetic)

Lumbar vertebrae
(parasympathetic)

Sacral vertebrae
(parasympathetic)

S2
S3
S4

C1
C2
C3
C4
C5
C6
C7
T1
T2
T3
T4
T5
T6
T7
T8
T9
T10
T11
T12
L1
L2
L3
L4
L5
S1
S2
S3
S4

The Role of the Autonomic Nervous System

The autonomic nervous system establishes the connection between the constituent parts of the body. Its two complementary parts ensure the maintenance of life by regulating nutrition, metabolism, and adaptation. Because of the opposing actions of these two parts, all disease stems from an imbalance in this system.

The sympathetic and the parasympathetic systems act on cellular permeability. The sympathetic system increases permeability, which in turn increases the number of cellular exchanges. This process, which raises basic metabolism and causes the body's reserves to melt down, is catabolic. The parasympathetic system reduces permeability, which lowers basic metabolism and increases the body's reserves. This anabolic process ensures the body's ability to sustain life.

In the embryo, the autonomic nervous system appears before the central nervous system during the fourth and fifth weeks of gestation. It regulates internal functions that are not subject to the will, such as those of the visceral organs, vessels, and glands.

It regulates the inner environment and brings about homeostasis through vascularization and glandular secretions. It protects the body from various kinds of attacks and ensures the functioning of its self-defense, self-regulating, and self-repairing abilities. It also regulates libido and blood pressure.

The Central Nervous System

The central nervous system consists of the brain, the spinal cord, and the rachidian nerves. Each rachidian nerve innervates one specific segment of the skin called a dermatome, which transmits sensory information to the rachidian nerves or to a segment of the spinal cord. The central nervous system governs the coordination of all impulses, no matter their point of origin.

The Peripheral Nervous System

The peripheral nervous system consists of the sensitive motor nerves that allow conscious perception and voluntary movements to exist.

The Dermatomes

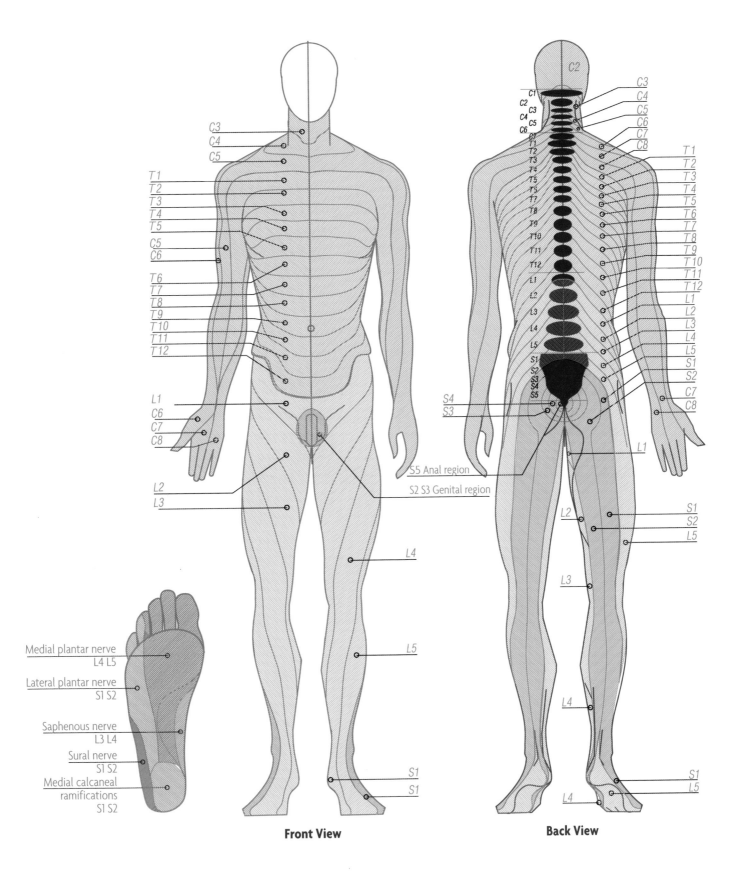

Front View

Medial plantar nerve
L4 L5

Lateral plantar nerve
S1 S2

Saphenous nerve
L3 L4

Sural nerve
S1 S2

Medial calcaneal
ramifications
S1 S2

S5 Anal region

S2 S3 Genital region

Back View

The Three Brains

The human brain consists of three main sections: the reptilian brain, the limbic brain, and the neocortex.

The reptilian brain is the oldest; it is the brain of the most primitive instincts. First appearing some five hundred million years ago, it still exists in *Homo sapiens*. It consists of the part of the central nervous system that goes from the brain stem to the hypothalamus. It integrates physiological data to allow the reception of basic information and generates responses necessary to survival and the perpetuation of the species.

The limbic brain appeared in the oldest mammals about three million years ago. Connected to the hypothalamus and the cerebral cortex, it refines the functions of the reptilian brain.

The limbic brain is involved with the primary emotions and the behaviors originating from them. It analyzes needs, governs impulses, and enables emotional responses to adapt to changes in the environment. It contributes to the maintenance of biochemical equilibrium and distributes electric and endocrinologic messages. It affects the duration of both sleeping and waking states.

The neocortex is made up of the cerebral hemispheres and is the headquarters for logical and conceptual thought. It integrates all intellectual data.

Handling the information that comes in from the outside world by means of the sense organs and the process of memory, the neocortex provides the necessary responses, intellectual and motor, to meet the demands of the ever-changing environment. It makes possible the functions of learning and selection—in a word, discrimination.

It stores in biochemical form the experiences selected by the limbic brain. It plays a role in all conscious and unconscious behaviors.

The left hemisphere of the neocortex is analytical and sees things from the particular to the whole. The right hemisphere is systemic and intuitive and proceeds from the whole to the particular. Appropriate thought, reflection, speech, and action depend upon effective exchange of information between the two hemispheres. This exchange takes place via the corpus callosum, which connects the two.

Reflexology of the Brain

The big toes reflect the entirety of the brain: the neocortex, the limbic and reptilian systems, the hippocampus, the amygdalae, the emotional relays, and the mammillary tubercles. The right hemisphere is mirrored on the right foot and the left hemisphere on the left foot.

On the big toe, when treating the zones concerned with memory problems, the pia mater, the dura mater, the arachnoid, the falx cerebri, and the tentorium cerebelli are addressed. (See pages 128 and 129.) This treatment activates blood circulation, as well as the circulation of lymph and CSF. The increased circulation then transmits impulses to the brain, which in turn acts upon all functions affected.

The thumbs also reflect the entirety of the brain. On the thumb, if a practitioner works the brain membranes, the dura mater, the pia mater, and the arachnoid, then the falx cerebri and the tentorium cerebelli, this effectively mitigates Alzheimer's disease, as well as improves memory function and diminishes phobias, among other things.

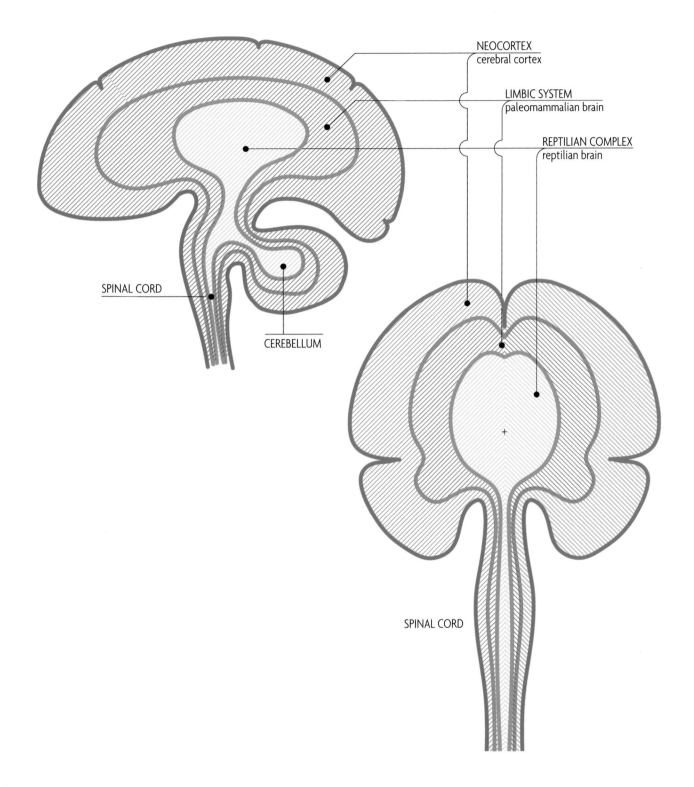

NEOCORTEX
cerebral cortex

LIMBIC SYSTEM
paleomammalian brain

REPTILIAN COMPLEX
reptilian brain

SPINAL CORD

CEREBELLUM

SPINAL CORD

The Plexuses

Energetic nervous centers, the seven plexuses are a kind of crossroads where the nerves are brought together. These seven centers correspond with the seven chakras and connect the three levels of being (mental, emotional, and physical) through the brain, the endocrine glands, and the cells.

The seven plexuses correspond with the three levels of being as follows: The coccygeal and the hypogastric plexuses reflect the physical level; the solar (or digestive) plexus, the cardiac plexus, and the thyroid plexus reflect the emotional level; and the pituitary (or hypophyseal) plexus and the pineal (or coronal) plexus reflect the mental level. (See pages 144 to 146 for more about the three levels of being.)

The Coccygeal Plexus

This plexus is located below the pubis, and its reflex point on the foot is situated in the center of the lower section of the calcaneus. It is the seat of procreation, growth, and sexuality. It is the manifestation of the human being's physical form and individual consciousness.

Attachment to earthly objects and the fear of losing them correspond to this plexus. Indeed, this is where energy becomes rooted, takes on material form, and then ascends to the brain.

The coccygeal plexus is ruled by the element of water. The very essence of life that constitutes three-fourths of the human being's body weight, water immerses the individual in tides (like the menstrual cycle) just as the moon influences the tides of the oceans. It is logical that this plexus should correspond to procreation, along with the gonads, ovaries, and testicles—all that embodies the life force.

The Hypogastric Plexus

This plexus is located two fingers' width below the navel, and its reflex point on the foot can be found on the upper inner edge of the calcaneus. It is the seat of elimination and excretion. It is also the seat of creative inspiration. Bones, hair, and nails draw their energy from the hypogastric plexus. Its corresponding glands are the adrenal glands.

The Solar (or Digestive) Plexus

This plexus is located above the navel, and its reflex point is located in the center of the foot. It is the seat of fear and anxiety. The solar plexus rules digestion and corresponds to the pancreas and the liver.

The Cardiac Plexus

This plexus is located at the level of vertebra T4, and its reflex point can be found above the center of the foot. This plexus is home to the connection between the body and the mind. The first to be affected by stress and mental attitudes, the cardiac plexus is the center of protection for the body and the immune system. It directs growth, muscular strength, and the circulation of lymph. It corresponds to the thymus.

The Thyroid Plexus

Corresponding with the thyroid, this plexus is situated in front of the trachea, and its reflex point is at the base of the first phalanx of the big toe. It is connected with oral expression.

Right Sole of Foot

Left Sole of Foot

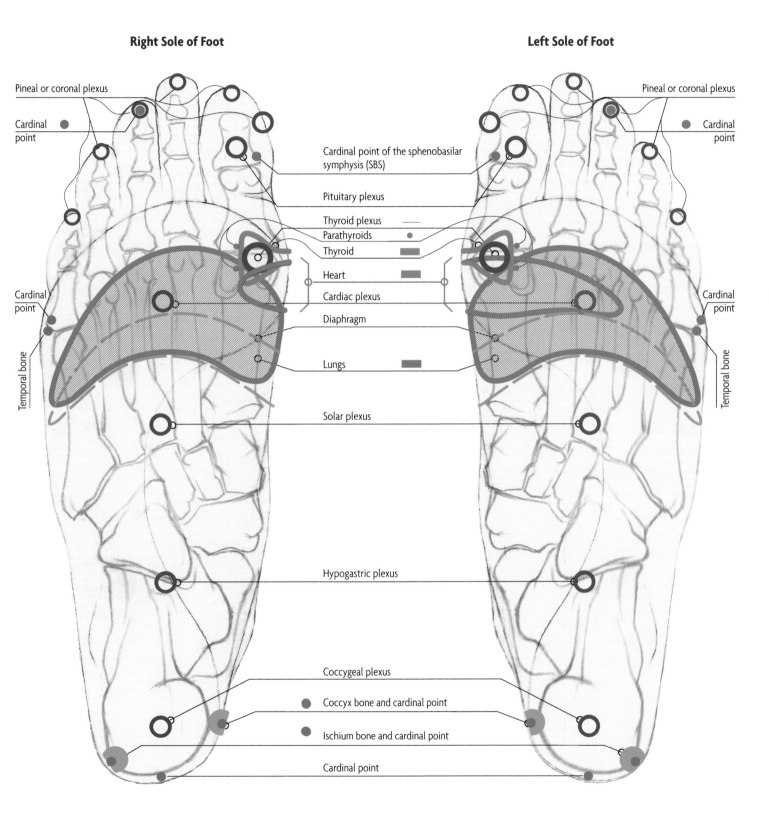

Pineal or coronal plexus

Cardinal point

Cardinal point

Temporal bone

Pineal or coronal plexus

Cardinal point

Cardinal point

Temporal bone

Cardinal point of the sphenobasilar symphysis (SBS)

Pituitary plexus

Thyroid plexus

Parathyroids

Thyroid

Heart

Cardiac plexus

Diaphragm

Lungs

Solar plexus

Hypogastric plexus

Coccygeal plexus

Coccyx bone and cardinal point

Ischium bone and cardinal point

Cardinal point

The Pituitary (or Hypophyseal) Plexus

The pituitary plexus is located in the center of the forehead, and its reflex point is found in the middle of the second phalanx of the big toe. It controls body fluids, such as blood and water. It corresponds to the pituitary gland and the hypothalamus.

The Pineal (or Coronal) Plexus

This plexus is located in the center of the head, and its reflex point is located on the outside edge of the big toe (above the points for the pituitary gland and the hypothalamus). More reflex points can also be found, like those of the pineal gland, on the top portions of the other toes. As the contact point between the endocrine system and the nervous system, the pineal gland sends hormones to the pituitary gland and the hypothalamus.

Interconnection of the Plexuses

The plexuses are connected by blood, lymph, the autonomic nervous system, and, first and foremost, the cerebrospinal fluid, which moves from the spinal column into the connective tissues to bathe the cells of the body. It stimulates these cells and transmits information to them.

Treatment of the Plexuses in Reflexology

Through treatment on the appropriate reflex points on the feet, reflexology works on the plexuses as follows:

1. In the coccygeal plexus, reflexology can help to regulate growth, sexuality (especially in the event of sterility), and disrupted menstrual cycles.
2. In the hypogastric plexus, it relieves pain and inflammation and improves elimination.
3. In the solar (or digestive) plexus, it treats diabetes and hypoglycemia and improves digestion and the metabolism of fats and sugars.
4. In the cardiac plexus, it addresses edema, the muscles, and circulation. It also stimulates the immune system.
5. In the thyroid plexus, it regulates disrupted metabolism and treats spasmophilia, osteoporosis, arthrosis, and arthritis.
6. In the pituitary (or hypophyseal) plexus, it addresses the hormonal system.
7. In the pineal (or coronal) plexus, it contributes to the repair of any disorders in the realm of the pineal gland.

Applying deep pressure on these reflex points rebalances plexus function, thereby helping to regulate the hormonal, immune, lymphatic, and craniosacral systems. By balancing these systems, reflexology can help to reestablish homeostasis.

The Chakras

Sahasrara

Ajna

Vishuddha

Anahata

Manipura

Svadhisthana

Muladhara

The Plexuses

Pineal

Pituitary

Thyroid

Cardiac

Solar

Hypogastric

Coccygeal

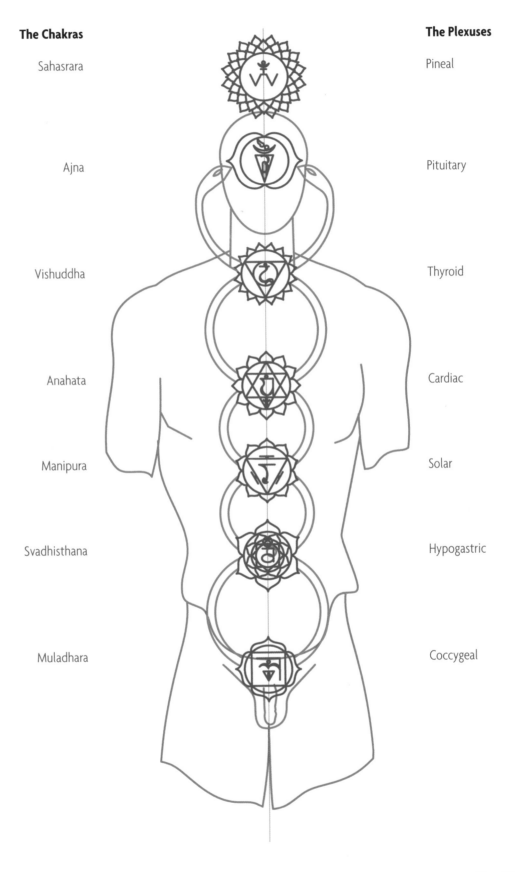

The Endocrine Glands and the Hormones

The nervous and endocrine systems regulate body functions such as metabolism, the internal cellular terrain (circulation, temperature, electrolytic balance, pH), growth, maturation, and reproduction. They coordinate the body's responses to the demands made upon it by the external environment. Whereas the nervous system transmits rapid signals of short duration through the nerves, the endocrine system relays its messages with hormones in a more prolonged journey through the circulatory system—it works more slowly than the nervous system but covers greater distances. Reflexology on the glandular and hormonal areas of the feet can help to balance and regulate these vital systems.

Synthesized by the endocrine glands, each of which resonates with a particular plexus, hormones are transported by the blood into the cells, where they are recognized by specific receptors. The endocrine glands form a system of oversight and command in the physiology of the body from its cells to its central nervous system. Recent studies have revealed the intimate relationship among the brain, the endocrine glands, and the immune system. This is why stress can lead to both a depressed immune system and psychological depression.

Each organ possesses a specific energetic frequency. Gathered together in the same region of the body, organs sharing the same frequency are also connected by a physiological relationship. That's why it's so important to understand the molecule as a vibratory energetic complex.

Hormones, enzymes, and other biochemical composites know which receptor they need to adapt to; even molecules appear to have the capacity to choose among the different reference points. The body can instantaneously produce hundreds of different chemical agents and govern their movements for the collective good of the whole.

The Endocrine Glands

As mentioned above, there is a very close relationship between the nervous system and the endocrine glands. They work in synergy to create homeostasis.

The Pineal Gland

The vestige of a third eye among certain migratory birds, the pineal gland is a third receptor of light located beneath the skin. It is literally a third eye because it consists of cells identical to those of the retina and informs the human being of external conditions of light and dark. It governs the endocrine cycle, which directs all body functions. It is the body's internal workings that bring about its adaptation to the external environment.

The pineal gland is shaped like a cone, weighs roughly sixteen grams, and is immersed in CSF. Located behind the limbic brain, it records the messages arriving from other parts of the brain and, thanks to the secretion of melatonin, which stimulates all the other hormones, it helps the glands respond to these messages.

The Pituitary Gland

About the size of a pea, the pituitary gland weighs about 0.5 gram. With the hypothalamus, it transmits hormonal stimulations to the other glands. This gland was long believed to be the master gland, but it is now known that the secretions of the pineal gland are the true regulators of the pituitary.

The Hypothalamus

The hypothalamus is a relay center that connects the pineal plexus and the pituitary plexus. Bathed in CSF, it analyzes, balances, and transforms energy. It controls the autonomic nervous system, body temperature, and

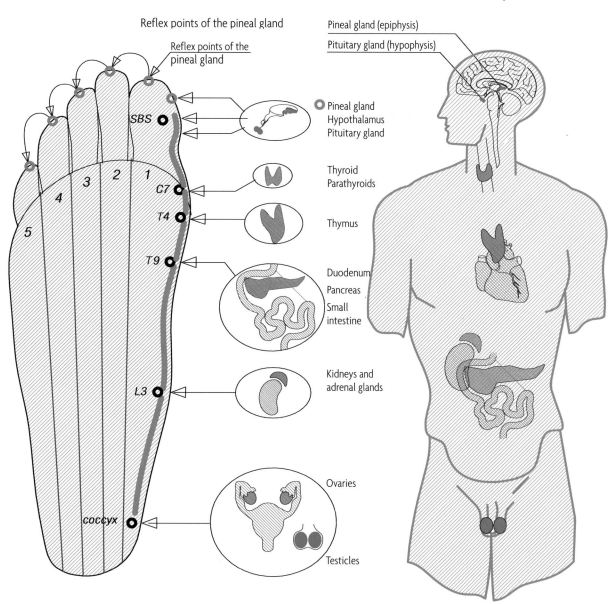

Reflex points of the pineal gland

Reflex points of the pineal gland

SBS

C7

T4

T9

L3

coccyx

1 2 3 4 5

Pineal gland (epiphysis)
Pituitary gland (hypophysis)

Pineal gland
Hypothalamus
Pituitary gland

Thyroid
Parathyroids

Thymus

Duodenum
Pancreas
Small
intestine

Kidneys and
adrenal glands

Ovaries

Testicles

the balance of fluids in the body. The hypothalamus also regulates any growth set forth by HGH (human growth hormone).

The Thyroid and the Parathyroids

The thyroid, which controls basic metabolism and cardiac rhythm, manages our abilities to adapt. It secretes thyroxine and needs the iodide contained in food to function properly. The thyroid enables the body to tol-

erate changes in the environment, from fluctuations in temperature to struggles with a new language to emotional difficulties. It works as a catalyst in the realms of emotion and communication. With the ovaries and the adrenal glands, it oversees the body's energy levels and energy production. This role can be abused when the body is affected by stress syndrome; the thyroid handles the body's increased need for energy and works harder to help it adapt to external changes.

The parathyroid glands play a major role in the absorption and fixation of calcium and phosphates. They accomplish this task through the secretion of parathormone, with the aid of ultraviolet light and vitamin D.

The Thymus

The thymus is a lymphatic organ located right in front of and above the heart. It develops fairly rapidly from the time of birth to puberty, then begins to shrink in volume. At the onset of adulthood, this organ goes to sleep, but resumes its function during the production of antibodies or whenever it is needed to oversee the immune system. Because of this role, its reflex zone is extremely important.

The Pancreas

A gland of mixed nature, both endocrine and exocrine, it produces two major hormones, insulin and glucagon (hyperglycemic factor). The balance between these two hormones must always remain stable at 80 percent insulin and 20 percent glucagon.

The Liver

The liver acts as a filter for the blood. This gland is also both endocrine and exocrine; it has glycogenic and ureopoietic action. It stores fats and is hematopoietic (involved in the production of blood cells). It produces the bile that is stored in the gallbladder. The liver consists mostly of water (97 percent) but also contains mineral salts, organic cholesterol composites, phospholipids, biliary salts, and bilirubin. Because of the phospholipids and biliary salts it contains, cholesterol that is insoluble in water becomes soluble in the bile contained in the liver and gallbladder.

The liver plays a role in various aspects of blood coagulation with the formation of fibrinogen and the absorption of vitamin K. It is bile that makes this possible, as it is essential for the synthesis of prothrombin and the manufacture of heparin (both of which assist in the process of coagulation).

The Adrenal Glands

The adrenal glands are made up of two entities that are endocrine in nature: the adrenal cortex and the adrenal medulla.

The adrenal cortex produces a cholinergic chemical transmitter and numerous hormones, including the corticosteroids. This group includes the mineralcorticosteroids, such as aldosterone, which governs the balance between sodium salts and potassium salts by retaining sodium.

The adrenal cortex also produces glucocorticoids and sex hormones. The glucocorticoids reduce the consumption of glucose in the cells and increase glycemia. They lower the number of lymphocytes in the blood and reduce inflammation. They also determine the level of resistance the body can produce in response to situations of stress (hunger, thirst, change in temperature). The androgens (male hormones) form from the synthesis and breakdown of corticoids. Female sex hormones (estrogen and progesterone) are formed in lesser quantity.

The adrenergic adrenal medulla is derived from sympathoblast cells and constitutes a sympathetic paraganglion. It also produces the hormones noradrenaline and adrenaline, which are chemical transmitters for postganglionary sympathetic neurons, part of the sympathetic nervous system.

The Mammary Glands

The mammary glands manufacture prolactin.

The Ovaries

Estrogen and progesterone are secreted primarily by the ovaries. The placenta, appearing during pregnancy, also secretes these hormones.

Estrogen experiences two principal peaks, one just before ovulation and one midway between ovulation and the onset of menstruation. It maintains and develops the female sexual organs, encourages tissue growth, and stimulates cell division, especially within the mucosal layers of the mouth, the nose, the skin, the uterus, and the mammary glands. It encourages calcification of the

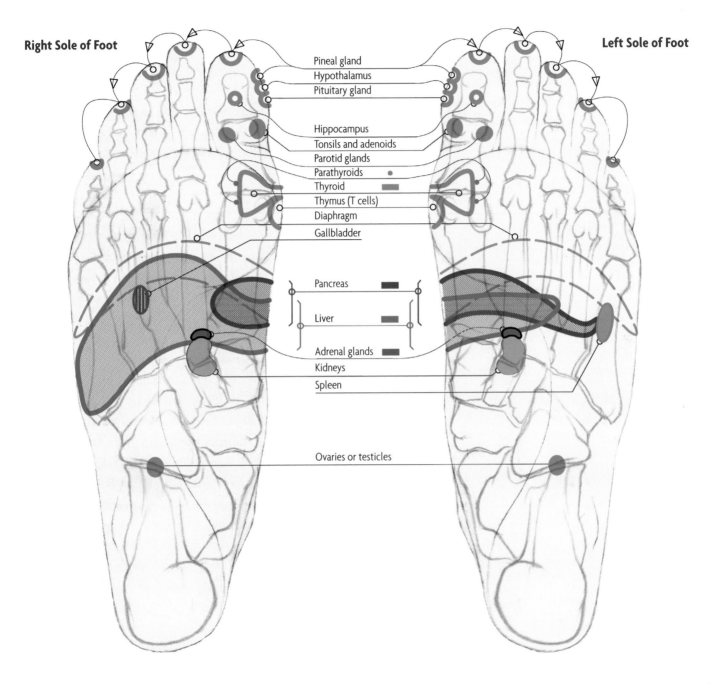

Right Sole of Foot

Left Sole of Foot

Pineal gland
Hypothalamus
Pituitary gland

Hippocampus
Tonsils and adenoids
Parotid glands
Parathyroids
Thyroid
Thymus (T cells)
Diaphragm
Gallbladder

Pancreas

Liver

Adrenal glands
Kidneys
Spleen

Ovaries or testicles

bones. Estrogen generates retention of water and salt; weight increase follows. It make the secretions of the sebaceous glands more fluid and inhibits them during an outbreak of acne. It brings down cholesterol levels in the blood and inhibits the formation of arteriosclerosis.

Progesterone is secreted by the corpus luteum of the ovaries. Its role is to transform the mucous membrane that has been highly developed by estrogen and make it more receptive to possible fertilization and the favorable development of the ovum.

The Testicles

These glands produce androgens, testosterone in particular, as well as minute quantities of female hormones.

Some Other Important Hormones

Adrenocorticotropic Hormone (ACTH)

This is the stress hormone. Secreted by the pituitary gland, ACTH triggers the release by the corticoadrenal glands of various glucocorticoids, especially cortisol. Along with adrenalin, it stimulates the breakdown of the glycogen stored in the liver and muscles into glucose, as well as the breakdown of the triglycerides found in the adipose tissues into glycerol and fatty acids. Once these elements have been broken down, they enter the bloodstream, providing a source of energy for use by the tissues. Cortisol triggers the breakdown of proteins, releasing amino acids that the body uses for the repair of lesions.

Growth Hormone

This hormone is secreted by the pituitary gland and completes the reparative action of cortisol. Seventy-five percent of the quantity of growth hormone secreted in a twenty-four-hour period is released at night, during deep and slow-wave sleep states.

Prolactin

The secretion of prolactin, another pituitary hormone, increases at the end of pregnancy, stimulating the production of milk by the mammary glands. It also plays a role in cellular division, reproduction, immunity, and sexual behavior.

Thyroid Stimulating Hormone (TSH)

Secreted by the pituitary gland in response to stimulation from the hypothalamus, TSH controls the regulation of body temperature. It triggers the thyroid to release hormones that increase heat production by oxidizing nutrients in the cells.

Insulin

Insulin is a digestive hormone that is secreted by the cells of the pancreas to stimulate the absorption of glucose by the cells. This glucose is then either stored in the form of glycogen or triglycerides or transformed into energy.

Glucagon

Glucagon is also secreted by the pancreas. It increases blood sugar levels by increasing the rate at which the liver breaks down stored sugar. It acts on the absorption of amino acids by the cells and on their transformation into proteins.

The Renin-Angiotensin System

This system controls arterial blood pressure. When blood pressure goes down, the kidneys release renin, which enters the bloodstream and stimulates the liver to produce angiotensin. The angiotensin then reduces the diameter of the arteries (vasoconstriction), thereby raising arterial blood pressure. Angiotensin encourages the adrenal glands to release aldosterone, which increases the reabsorption of water and sodium by the kidneys. This process causes blood pressure to rise. The control of the secretion of renin is dependent upon the concentration of sodium in the blood, arterial blood pressure, and the action of the sympathetic nervous system.

Right Sole of Foot

Left Sole of Foot

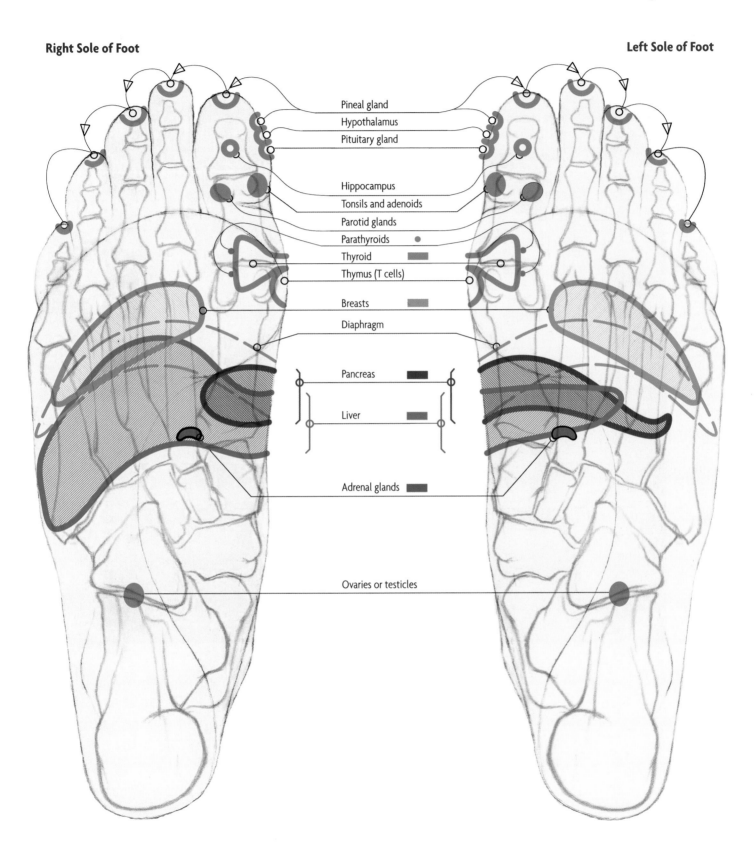

Pineal gland

Hypothalamus

Pituitary gland

Hippocampus

Tonsils and adenoids

Parotid glands

Parathyroids

Thyroid

Thymus (T cells)

Breasts

Diaphragm

Pancreas

Liver

Adrenal glands

Ovaries or testicles

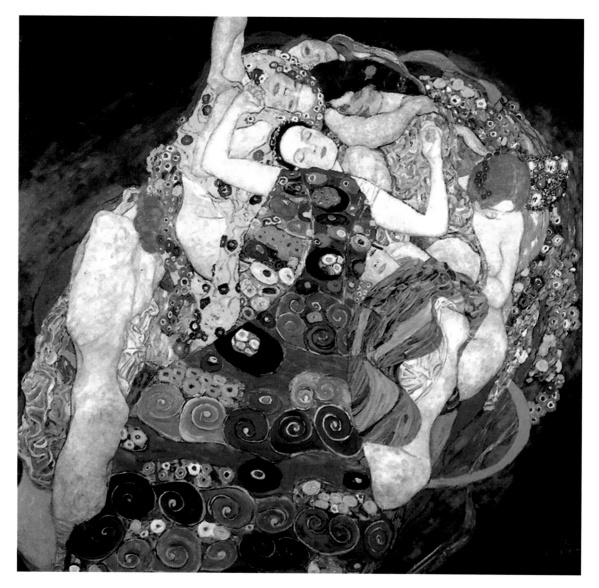

The Virgins, *by Gustav Klimt, 1913*
Narodni Gallery

(PHOTO ROGER VIOLLET)

Sleep

Sleep unfolds in successive cycles, each around ninety minutes in length. Each cycle includes a phase of slow-wave sleep followed by a phase of rapid eye movement (REM) sleep. This same rhythm governs the fluctuations of numerous hormones.

During the phase of waking directly preceding sleep, the hormones necessary for falling asleep are being manufactured. The systems controlling waking are then turned down. Waking and sleeping are both dependent upon the interaction of anatomical and biochemical factors.

The hypothalamus plays a key role in the phenomenon of going to sleep. When its posterior part is activated, the body is maintained in the waking state. When the anterior part is activated, the posterior aspect is inhibited, and sleep settles in.

The dorsal raphe nucleus (on the median line of the brain stem) comes into play during the onset of sleep by releasing serotonin. The basal nucleus of Meynert controls slow-wave sleep.

Rapid Eye Movement Sleep

REM sleep is directed by structures located within the lower brain stem and through the interaction of several neuronal systems. Circadian rhythm (the roughly twenty-four-hour cycle in the biochemical, physiological, and behavioral processes of living beings) functions under the influence of an internal biological clock located in the hypothalamus. During REM sleep, oneiric (dream) activity occurs four or five times a night, lasting for fifteen to twenty minutes at a time.

Metabolic Variations of the Brain During Sleep

Independent of the neurotransmitters and the modulating peptides, there are certain cerebral metabolic variations that make it possible to explain the onset of sleep.

During periods of activity, the brain experiences the same energetic conditions as a muscle: the glucose consumption of the cortical areas doubles without any variation in the percentage of oxygen utilized. It is therefore functioning in an anaerobic state, producing lactates like a muscle in full effort.

During the course of slow-wave sleep, the brain's consumption of glucose diminishes by 20 to 40 percent, whereas during REM sleep it increases to the same levels as in the waking state.

Thermoregulation

In conjunction with the metabolizing of glucose and the consumption of oxygen, body temperature has a major influence over sleep and varies in accordance with the internal clock. At 4:00 PM it is at its maximum (37.5 Centigrade or 99.5 Fahrenheit) and at 4:00 AM, the period that corresponds to the peak of rapid eye movement sleep, it is at its minimum level (36.5 Centigrade or 98.6 Fahrenheit). Afterward, it rises again, and there is a secretion of hormones, including cortisol, which begin to prepare the body for waking up in about three hours.

Action of Neurotransmitters on Sleep

Acetylcholine has its maximal curve of release in the cerebral cortex during waking hours and is at its minimum during slow-wave sleep. Its synthesis is reactivated at the level of the brain stem during REM sleep, whose every stage it oversees.

Gamma-aminobutyric acid (GABA) is present almost everywhere in the brain and has an inhibitory function on neurons. Glycine is another inhibitory neurotransmitter and comes into play on the level of the spinal cord. Serotonin, which is crucial for the onset of sleep, is released during the waking state. Its action permits the synthesis of hypnogenic factors. Interleukins (secreted by the immune system) facilitate deep slow-wave sleep. The onset of slow-wave sleep lowers blood pressure and heart rhythm.

Hormonal Secretion and Sleep

The interaction of hormones with sleep may be due to the anatomical proximity of the control centers for sleep and hormones.

Human growth hormone is released during the first phase of a deep slow-wave sleep. Cortisol, which is produced by the adrenal glands, ACTH, which is produced by the pituitary gland, and melatonin, which is secreted by the pineal gland, are all produced in correspondence with circadian rhythm. Cortisol prevents the onset of deep sleep. Melatonin, which promotes sleep, has a weak rate of secretion by day and a strong rate by night, just before sleep settles in.

Prolactin, which is released by the pituitary gland during sleep, reaches its minimum stage during the day. Insulin production is dependent upon the cycle of waking and sleeping. Thyrotropin (thyroid-stimulating hormone, or TSH), produced by the pituitary gland, has a complex secretion cycle that is connected with both sleep and circadian rhythm. Its production goes down during deep sleep.

Renin, secreted by the kidneys, is also dependent upon sleep. Its phases of oscillation last ninety minutes, just like the cycles of sleep. Its production increases during deep sleep, then diminishes during slow-wave sleep. Waking up brings about an even further reduction.

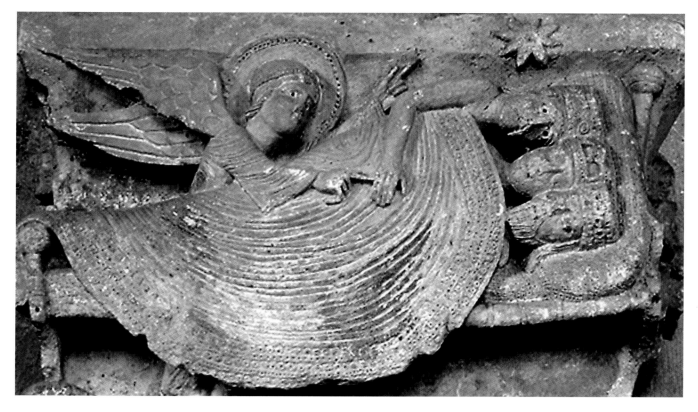

The Sleep of the Magi
Autun Cathedral

The Systems of the Body

In the following pages we shall review the principles of the following systems in succession, from both an anatomical standpoint and a consideration of overall health:

The diagrams on pages 67, 68, and 69 show the important points and zones of two or more systems overlaid with each other to show possible interactions and correspondences between systems.

---

*Note that because of its complexity, the lymphatic system will be discussed in a separate chapter unto itself; the first five systems listed here will be covered in this chapter.

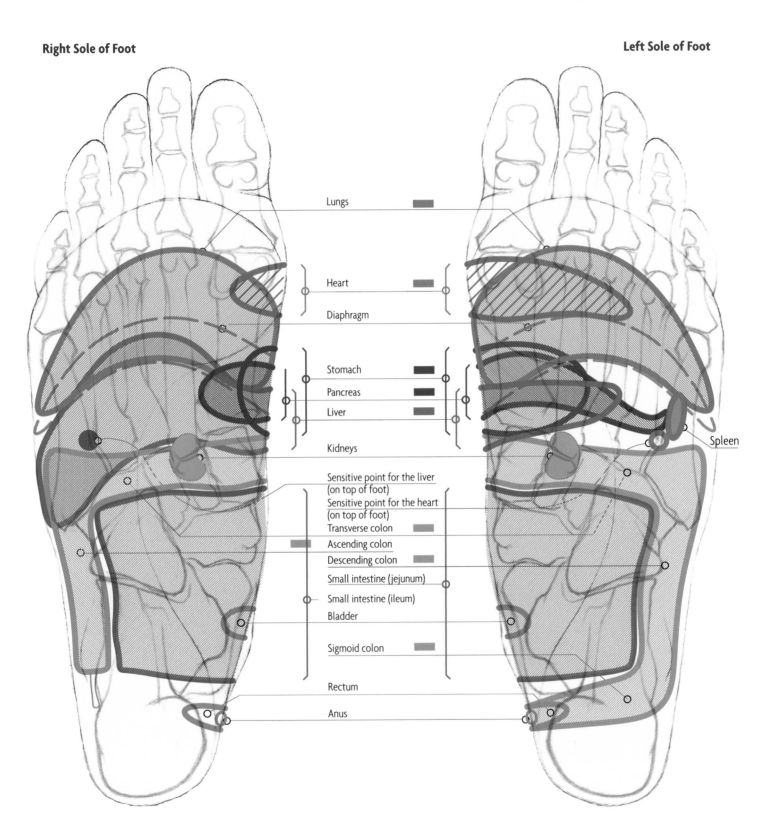

Right Sole of Foot

Left Sole of Foot

Lungs

Heart

Diaphragm

Stomach

Pancreas

Liver

Kidneys

Sensitive point for the liver
(on top of foot)
Sensitive point for the heart
(on top of foot)
Transverse colon

Ascending colon

Descending colon

Small intestine (jejunum)

Small intestine (ileum)

Bladder

Sigmoid colon

Rectum

Anus

Spleen

1. The Skeletal System

Because the skeleton is the foundation of the body, a person's standing posture can reveal a lot about his or her overall health. The skeleton experiences profound transformations over the course of an individual's life. It becomes more fragile during times of hormonal change (growth, puberty, and menopause).

The parathyroid glands, controlled by the liver, regulate the fixation of minerals in the bones, and the pituitary gland acts on bone growth.

The skeleton requires a balanced diet that includes vitamins C, D, and B; proper intestinal absorption; a healthy hormonal system; and regular physical activity, which stimulates the formation of bone cells. A deficient and acidic diet (sugars, tomatoes, citrus fruits, tea, coffee) is harmful to the bones, as is stress, because it inhibits the stomach and mucous membranes, hindering their ability to absorb minerals. Should this problem reach a crisis point, eliminate meats, processed lunch meats, fish, and dairy products from the diet in addition to the acidic foods listed above.

The Spine

The spine's complex construction makes it highly susceptible to certain injuries. Back pain, encouraged by a sedentary lifestyle, has become a common ailment. Massaging the zones of the spine on the feet relaxes the associated back muscles, alleviates pain, and, combined with a back-friendly lifestyle, is an excellent injury-preventive measure.

Locating the Spine Zones

The spine zones are located along the inner edges of the feet in the first zone (see page 55). The zone of the cervical spine runs along the first base joint. Next to it is the zone of the thoracic spine, which follows the outer edge of the first metatarsal bone. The transition from the base joint of the toe to the first metatarsal bone is the zone marking the point of transition from the neck to the chest part of the spine. The lumbar spine is represented in the area of the tarsal bones (the cuboid bone and the navicular bone). The sacrum is reflected on the inside rim of the heel.

The Spinal Column and the Inner Arch of the Foot

This depiction of the inner profile of the arch of the foot following the curve of the spinal column corresponds pretty closely to the actual reflex points. However, for the precise positions of the reflex points for each vertebra, refer to the side view at the bottom of this page or the plate The Vertebrae on the Arch of the Foot.

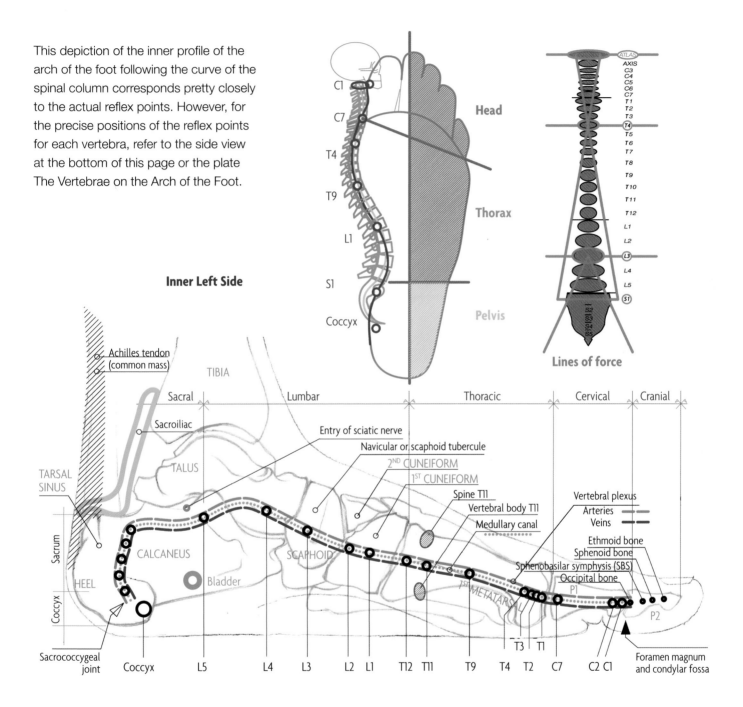

Inner Left Side

Head

Thorax

Pelvis

Lines of force

C1
C7
T4
T9
L1
S1
Coccyx

ATLAS
AXIS
C3
C4
C5
C6
C7
T1
T2
T3
T4
T5
T6
T7
T8
T9
T10
T11
T12
L1
L2
L3
L4
L5
S1
S2
S3
S4
S5

Achilles tendon (common mass)
TIBIA
Sacral
Sacroiliac
Entry of sciatic nerve
Navicular or scaphoid tubercule
Lumbar
Thoracic
Cervical
Cranial
2ND CUNEIFORM
1ST CUNEIFORM
Spine T11
Vertebral body T11
Medullary canal
Vertebral plexus
Arteries
Veins
Ethmoid bone
Sphenoid bone
Sphenobasilar symphysis (SBS)
Occipital bone
TALUS
TARSAL SINUS
Sacrum
CALCANEUS
SCAPHOID
Bladder
HEEL
Coccyx
1ST METATARSAL
P1
P2
Sacrococcygeal joint
Coccyx
L5
L4
L3
L2
L1
T12
T11
T9
T4
T3
T2
T1
C7
C2
C1
Foramen magnum and condylar fossa

The Spinal Column
Lines of Force

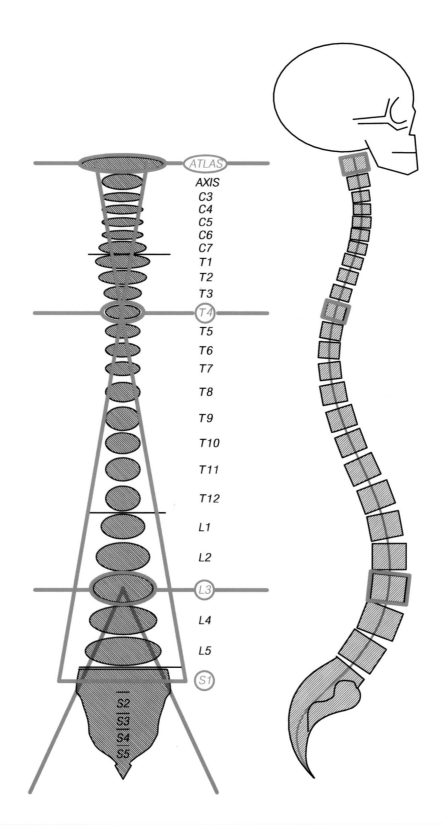

ATLAS
AXIS
C3
C4
C5
C6
C7
T1
T2
T3
T4
T5
T6
T7
T8
T9
T10
T11
T12
L1
L2
L3
L4
L5
S1
S2
S3
S4
S5

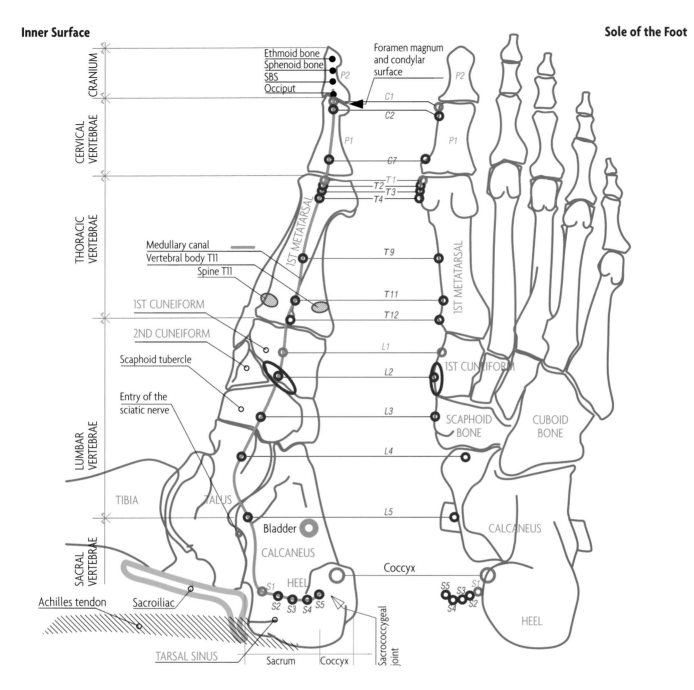

Inner Surface

Sole of the Foot

CRANIUM

CERVICAL VERTEBRAE

THORACIC VERTEBRAE

LUMBAR VERTEBRAE

SACRAL VERTEBRAE

Ethmoid bone
Sphenoid bone
SBS
Occiput

Foramen magnum and condylar surface

P2
C1
C2
P1
C7
T1
T2
T3
T4

1ST METATARSAL

Medullary canal
Vertebral body T11
Spine T11

T9
T11
T12
L1
L2
L3
L4
L5

1ST CUNEIFORM
2ND CUNEIFORM
Scaphoid tubercle
Entry of the sciatic nerve

1ST METATARSAL

1ST CUNEIFORM

SCAPHOID BONE

CUBOID BONE

CALCANEUS

TIBIA
TALUS

Bladder
CALCANEUS
HEEL

Coccyx

S1
S2 S3 S4 S5

Achilles tendon
Sacroiliac

TARSAL SINUS

Sacrum

Coccyx

Sacrococcygeal joint

S5 S3 S1
S4 S2

HEEL

The therapist should pay close attention to the position of the vertebrae reflex points on the inner surface of the foot. The vertical projection of these points onto the sole is shown above. Note how the vertical projection of the sacral vertebrae points would simply yield a single pressure point in the sole diagram instead of the five that are depicted here in a purely conventional fashion. In the same way, L2 is located on the inner lateral surface of the arch of the foot,

on the edge of the first cuneiform bone at its border with the scaphoid bone; its projection on the sole, however, places it almost at the very center of the cuneiform bone—which is wrong. For this reason, I have depicted this important vertebra by both a point and a zone, best viewed here in the lateral diagram, with the projection on the sole shown as well.

2. The Digestive System

The digestive system manages the processes of digestion, food assimilation, and elimination. Essentially one long continuous tube that extends from the mouth to the anus, it is part of the body's external context, like the skin.

The sacral parasympathetic system controls the terminal part of the digestive tube (descending colon, rectum). Because of this connection to the parasympathetic nervous system, the origins for several digestive disorders can be traced back to imbalances in the autonomic nervous system.

The pneumogastric (or vagus) nerve innervates all the digestive organs. It ensures favorable conditions for the digestion and absorption of foods.

The pancreas digests carbohydrates, lipids, and protides (proteins and their hydrolysis products). It also has a hormonal function as the producer of insulin and glucagon.

The liver digests fats and processes the steroidal hormones, beginning with cholesterol. It metabolizes carbohydrates and governs the function of muscles and tendons. The mouth and the duodenum (the entry to the small intestine) transform simple carbohydrates into glucose.

The stomach transforms proteins into polypeptides. It then reabsorbs the iron. The duodenum and the jejunum (the first two fifths of the small intestine) break down the polypeptides into amino acids. Lipids are digested in three stages: first, the bile emulsifies the fats; second, the pancreas hydrolyzes them; third, the jejunum's mucous membrane absorbs them. The lymph plays the final role of transporting them through the thoracic duct to the liver.

The ileum (the final three fifths of the small intestine) absorbs vitamins B, C, H (biotin), and P (bioflavonoids). The small intestine and the colon absorb water and mineral salts. The jejunum absorbs calcium.

Locating the Reflex Zones of the Digestive System

The zone of the mouth cavity is located on the inner edge of the big toe. On the sole of the foot, the esophagus zone extends from the base joint of the big toe along the first metatarsal bone. On the left foot, it reaches the stomach zone. On the right foot, it is shorter, ending in the ball of the foot. The zones of the mouth cavity and the esophagus are also found on the tops of the feet, the mouth zone at the joint between the first and second big-toe bones, and the esophagus zone extending from the middle of the first big-toe bone into the top of the first metatarsal bone. The gallbladder zone is on the sole of the right foot at the base of the third metatarsal bone. The zone of the liver extends over both soles; the larger part is located on the right sole, along the breadth of the first four metatarsal bones. Below the liver zone are the zones for the pancreas and the stomach.

The zone of the digestive tract is represented on the soles of the feet. The stomach zone is found primarily on the left foot; it extends sideways over the base of the first two metatarsal bones. The zone of the large intestine, or colon, and its three components starts in the right foot on the base of the heel bone and runs toward the toes up to the base of the fourth metatarsal bone. It then turns right and runs across the left foot to the base of its fourth metatarsal bone. From here it runs downward to the heel bone and then back to the inner edge of the foot, where on both feet the rectum zone is located. The rectum zone extends to the outer edges of the heel bone. The large intestine zone thus to some degree frames the small intestine zone, which is located on both soles.

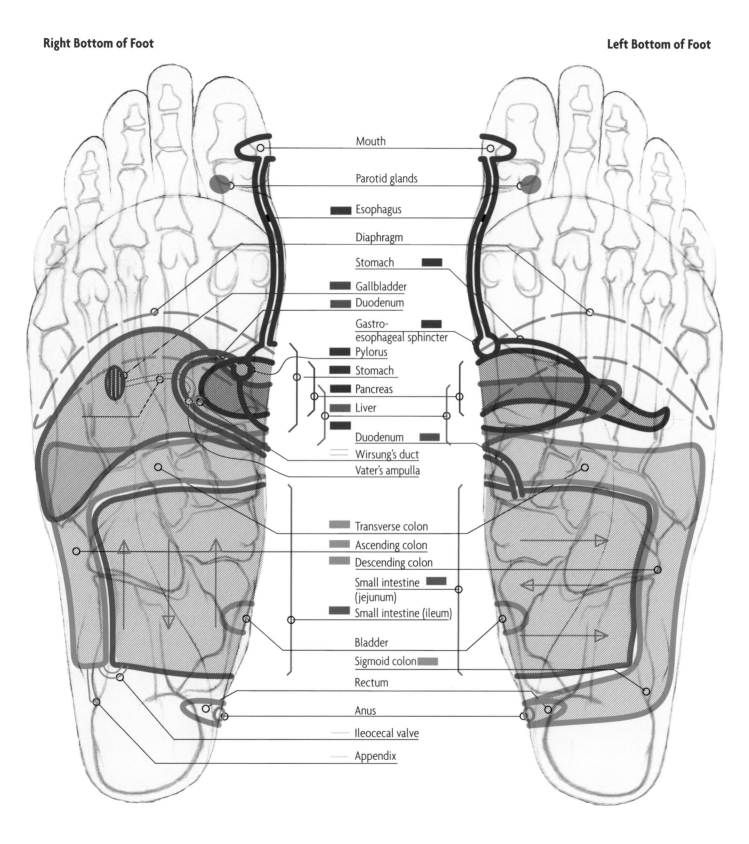

Right Bottom of Foot

Left Bottom of Foot

Mouth

Parotid glands

Esophagus

Diaphragm

Stomach

Gallbladder

Duodenum

Gastro-
esophageal sphincter

Pylorus

Stomach

Pancreas

Liver

Duodenum

Wirsung's duct

Vater's ampulla

Transverse colon

Ascending colon

Descending colon

Small intestine
(jejunum)

Small intestine (ileum)

Bladder

Sigmoid colon

Rectum

Anus

Ileocecal valve

Appendix

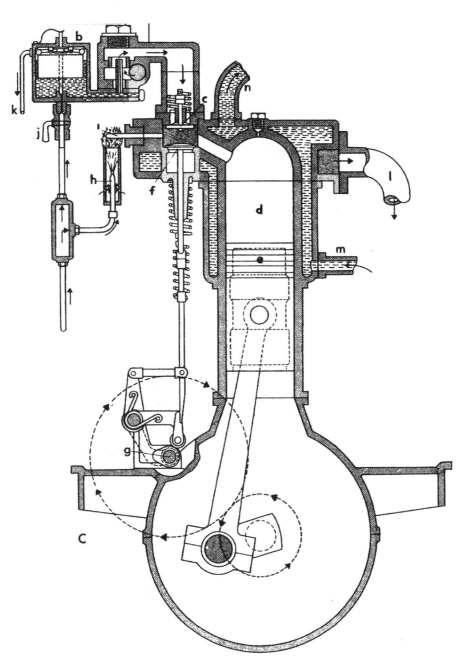

The urinary system is a machine . . .

3. The Urinary System

Made up of the kidneys, the ureters, the bladder, and the urethra, the urinary system produces, stores, and eliminates urine. The main actions of this system occur in the kidneys.

The kidneys help maintain the homeostatic balance of the body by filtering metabolites and minerals from the blood and excreting them, along with water, as urine. The kidneys filter approximately 180 liters of blood and produce around 1.5 liters of urine a day. They excrete urea and uric acid and store glucose and amino acids. They play a role in the synthesis of hormones and in the process of metabolism by transforming protides and peptides. They are involved in the production of bone marrow, red corpuscles, and the vitamin D necessary for the absorption of calcium.

Among the kidneys' homeostatic functions are maintenance of blood pH level, regulation of electrolyte concentrations, control of blood volume, and regulation of blood pressure. The kidneys accomplish their homeostatic functions independently and through coordination with other organs, particularly those of the endocrine system. The kidneys communicate with these organs through hormones secreted into the bloodstream.

The following symptoms may be evidence of a kidney (renal) disorder: lumbago on awakening that clears upon standing, overall morning fatigure, great thirst, muscle cramps, itching sensations in the lower limbs, fluctuations in blood pressure, pains beneath the heels, urinary problems, and dehydrated skin or darker skin tone.

Emotions have repercussions on the urinary system. Fear, for example, attacks the kidneys, and anxiety and strong emotions influence urination.

Locating the Reflex Zones of the Urinary Tract and Pelvic Organs

The kidney zone is shaped like the kidney itself. The zone is about the size of a bean and is located at the base of the third metatarsal bone. The zone of the ureter runs from the kidney zone across to the inside of the heel.

The bladder zone is about two finger-widths below the bottom edge of the ankle, toward the heel. Farther toward the heel is, in men, the zone of the sexual organs: the prostate, penis, and testicles. In women, the zone of the uterus is directly below the bladder zone but more toward the sole of the foot. The zone of the fallopian tube or vas deferens (seiminal duct) wraps around the top of the foot (see page 61).

The Urogenital System
Uterus/Prostate
Ovaries/Testicles

Right Sole of Foot

Left Sole of Foot

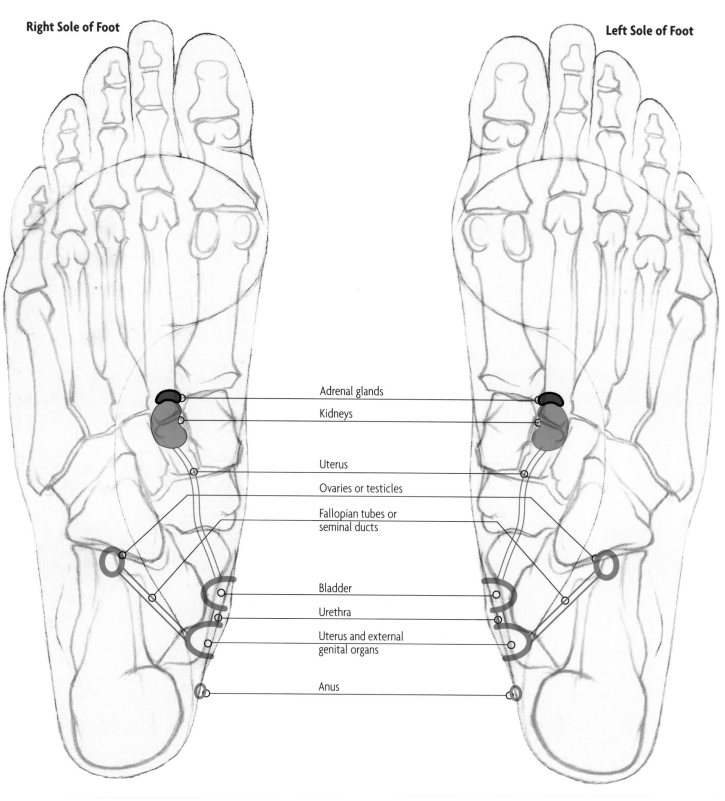

Adrenal glands

Kidneys

Uterus

Ovaries or testicles

Fallopian tubes or
seminal ducts

Bladder

Urethra

Uterus and external
genital organs

Anus

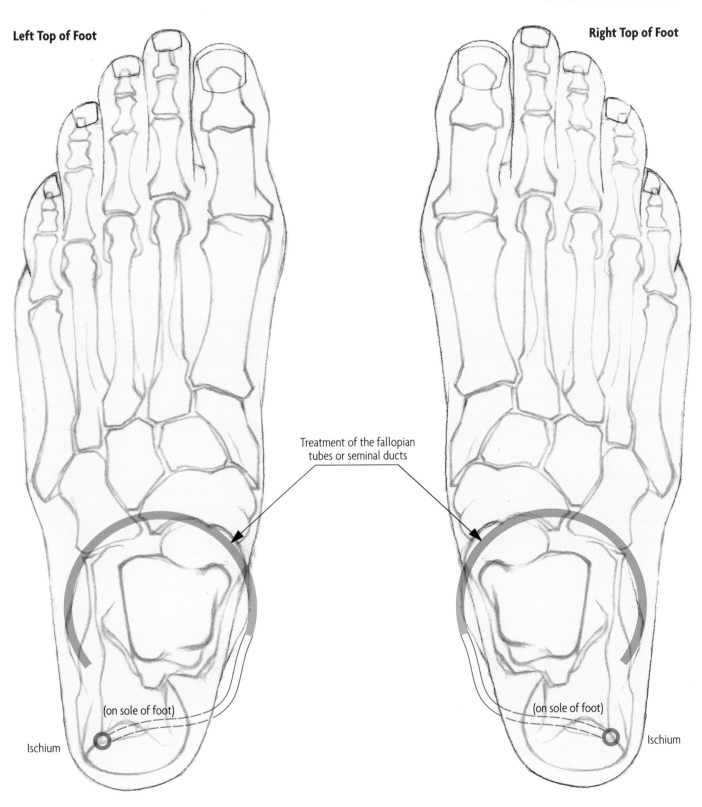

Left Top of Foot

Right Top of Foot

Treatment of the fallopian tubes or seminal ducts

(on sole of foot)

(on sole of foot)

Ischium

Ischium

4. The Respiratory System

The respiratory system consists of the sinuses, the airways, the lungs, and the respiratory muscles that control the movement of air into and out of the body.

The lungs ensure that proper oxygenation of the blood takes place by supplying oxygen and expelling carbon dioxide. The nasal fossae, the sinuses, the nasal cavity, and the pharynx warm up incoming air, then humidify and purify it before it reaches the alveoli in the lungs, where gaseous exchanges (O_2/CO_2) between air and blood take place. The lymphatic cells of the tonsils and the adenoids fight against viruses and bacteria that seek to enter the body by way of the mouth and the nose.

The nasal fossae consist of the frontal, ethmoidal, maxillary, and sphenoidal sinuses. If they are compressed during birth or, later on in life, by blows to the head, they can lose their mobility and air cannot circulate properly. The blocked mucous membranes lose their mucous covering and become vulnerable to microbes.

Blocked cranial sutures often provide a breeding ground for respiratory diseases: the nasal cavity becomes an enclosed culture medium responsible for digestive and respiratory infections. Respiratory catarrh comes in contact with food being swallowed; when this reaches the intestines, an inflammation occurs, particularly around the area of the ileocecal valve.

Dairy products, which are difficult to digest, irritate the intestinal mucous membrane, making it more vulnerable to catarrh that has been swallowed.

Infants are particularly vulnerable to ailments affecting the otolaryngological parts of the body (ear, nose, throat), as their sinuses are not yet sufficiently developed. When a mother nurses her baby, the child benefits from her immunities and thereby receives protection against infection.

Fear can alter the respiratory mucous membranes. Illnesses affecting the throat often point to unexpressed emotions felt in the stomach; a painful constriction (lump in the throat) results.

The increase in respiratory allergies today has a variety of possible origins: climate, pollution, animal dander, food preservatives, pollen, certain medications and vaccines, mold, and cow's milk. These allergens provoke an inflammatory reaction from the respiratory mucous membranes, accompanied by spasms and heavy secretion of catarrh.

Locating the Reflex Areas of the Cardiorespiratory System

The nose-throat zone extends from the front of the big toe around its base. The lung zone stretches across all five metatarsal bones. The trachea zone runs across the base joint of the big toe into the lung zone. The heart zone extends from the inside edge of the foot across the middle of the first metatarsal bone on the right foot and across the first, second, and third metatarsal bones on the left foot. The diaphragm zone runs along the middle of the metatarsal bones. Below the zone of the diaphragm is a large zone stretching to the heel corresponding to the abdominal muscles.

Right Sole of Foot

Left Sole of Foot

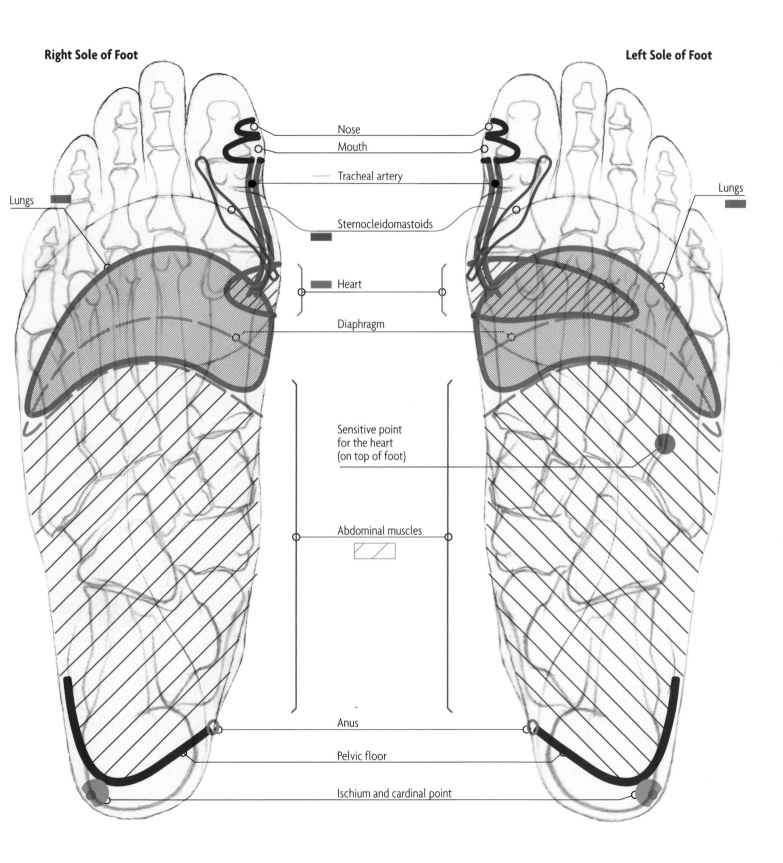

Nose

Mouth

Tracheal artery

Sternocleidomastoids

Lungs

Lungs

Heart

Diaphragm

Sensitive point
for the heart
(on top of foot)

Abdominal muscles

Anus

Pelvic floor

Ischium and cardinal point

5. The Circulatory System

The circulatory system consists of the heart, the blood, and the blood vessels. Blood circulation begins in the left atrium of the heart, where blood is pumped from the left ventricle through the arteries out to the capillaries of the organs and tissues. This blood returns via the veins to the right atrium of the heart: this completes one cycle of systemic circulation. From the right ventricle, the blood is pumped to the lungs for oxygenation, then circulated back to the left atrium: this completes one cycle of pulmonary circulation.

The heart beats approximately seventy times per minute, producing a cardiac output of some five liters per minute.

High Blood Pressure

Normal blood pressure for an adult at rest is 120/80. High blood pressure begins at about 140/90.

A distinction is made between emotional high blood pressure (when an increase is shown only in the top number of the reading) and true high blood pressure (when both the top and bottom figures of the reading are elevated above 140/90). True high blood pressure indicates peripheral resistance to arterial circulation that the heart must pump against.

Certain factors (stress, tobacco, overeating, birth control pills) in addition to high blood pressure set up the conditions for arteriosclerosis. High blood pressure can also have a hormonal or renal origin. When combined with tobacco, birth control pills can exacerbate high blood pressure.

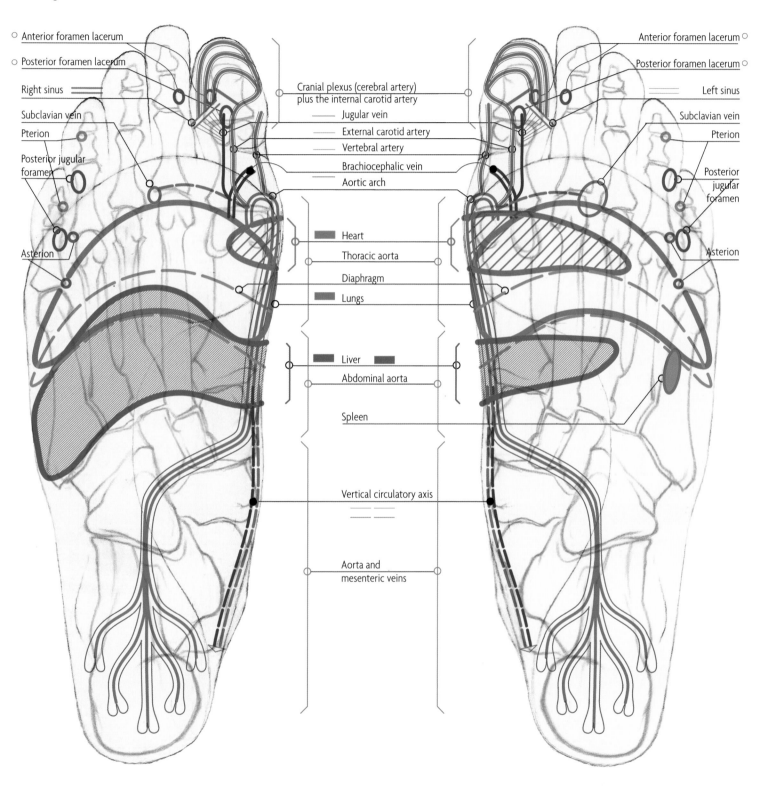

Right Sole of Foot

Left Sole of Foot

Anterior foramen lacerum

Posterior foramen lacerum

Right sinus

Subclavian vein

Pterion

Posterior jugular foramen

Asterion

Cranial plexus (cerebral artery) plus the internal carotid artery

Jugular vein

External carotid artery

Vertebral artery

Brachiocephalic vein

Aortic arch

Heart

Thoracic aorta

Diaphragm

Lungs

Liver

Abdominal aorta

Spleen

Vertical circulatory axis

Aorta and mesenteric veins

Anterior foramen lacerum

Posterior foramen lacerum

Left sinus

Subclavian vein

Pterion

Posterior jugular foramen

Asterion

The Circulatory System
Front View

The Arteries

The Veins

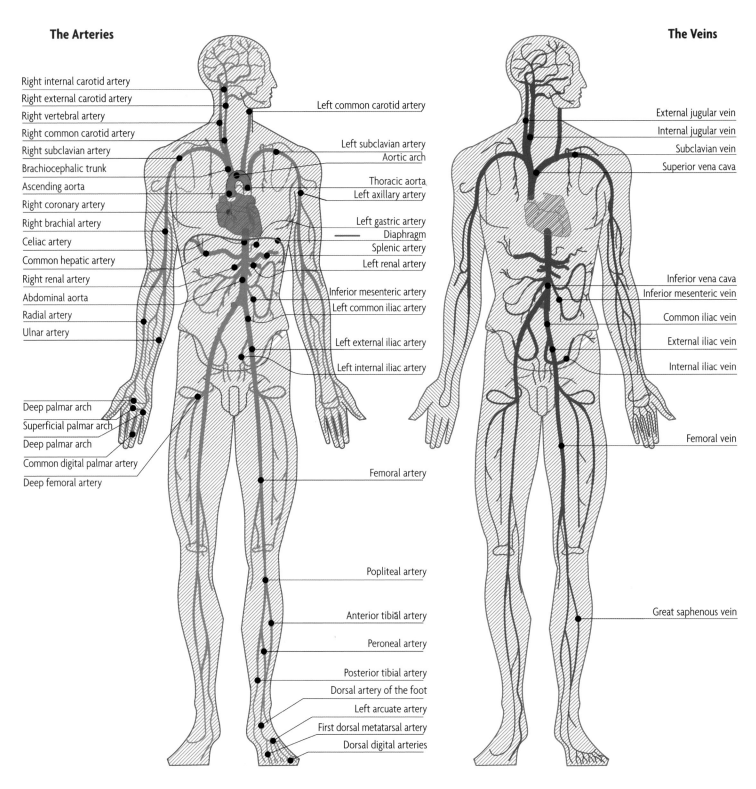

Right internal carotid artery
Right external carotid artery
Right vertebral artery
Right common carotid artery
Right subclavian artery
Brachiocephalic trunk
Ascending aorta
Right coronary artery
Right brachial artery
Celiac artery
Common hepatic artery
Right renal artery
Abdominal aorta
Radial artery
Ulnar artery

Deep palmar arch
Superficial palmar arch
Deep palmar arch
Common digital palmar artery
Deep femoral artery

Left common carotid artery

Left subclavian artery
Aortic arch

Thoracic aorta
Left axillary artery

Left gastric artery
Diaphragm
Splenic artery
Left renal artery

Inferior mesenteric artery
Left common iliac artery

Left external iliac artery

Left internal iliac artery

Femoral artery

Popliteal artery

Anterior tibial artery

Peroneal artery

Posterior tibial artery
Dorsal artery of the foot
Left arcuate artery
First dorsal metatarsal artery
Dorsal digital arteries

External jugular vein
Internal jugular vein
Subclavian vein
Superior vena cava

Inferior vena cava
Inferior mesenteric vein

Common iliac vein

External iliac vein

Internal iliac vein

Femoral vein

Great saphenous vein

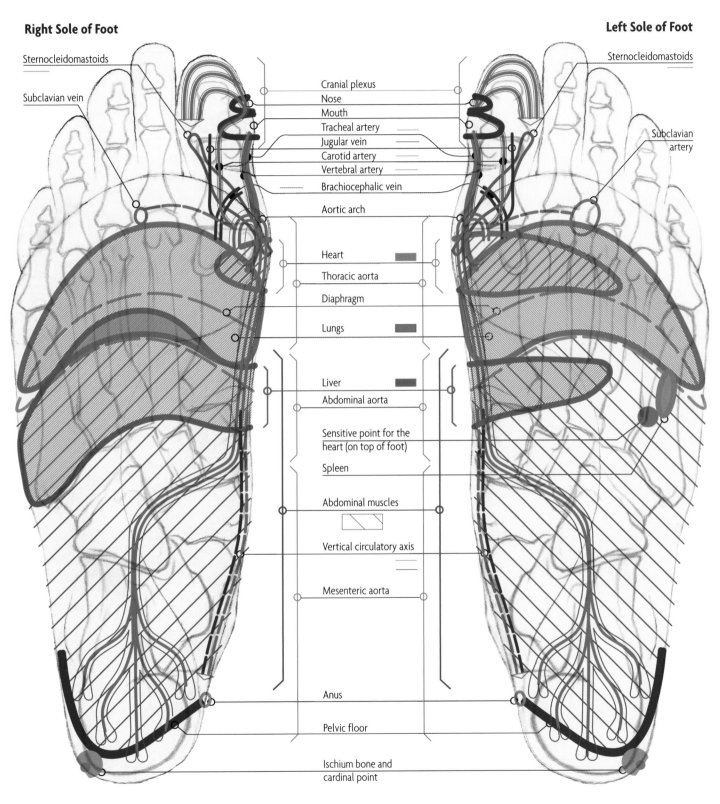

Right Sole of Foot

Left Sole of Foot

Sternocleidomastoids

Subclavian vein

Sternocleidomastoids

Subclavian artery

Cranial plexus
Nose
Mouth
Tracheal artery
Jugular vein
Carotid artery
Vertebral artery
Brachiocephalic vein

Aortic arch

Heart

Thoracic aorta

Diaphragm

Lungs

Liver
Abdominal aorta

Sensitive point for the heart (on top of foot)

Spleen

Abdominal muscles

Vertical circulatory axis

Mesenteric aorta

Anus

Pelvic floor

Ischium bone and cardinal point

Synthesis of the Hormonal, Digestive, and General Organ Systems with the Plexuses

Right Sole of Foot

Left Sole of Foot

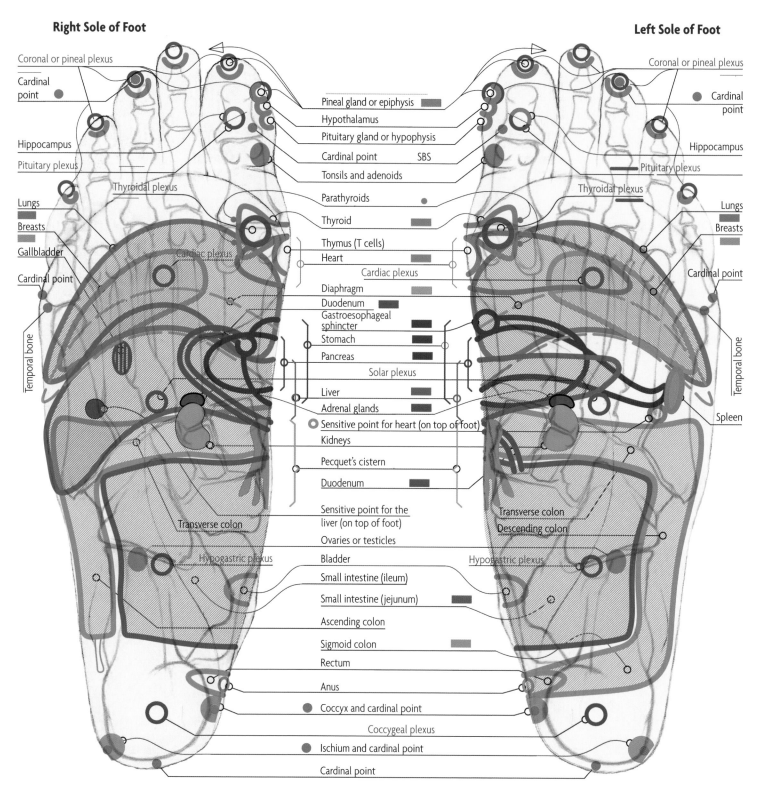

Coronal or pineal plexus

Cardinal point

Hippocampus

Pituitary plexus

Thyroidal plexus

Lungs

Breasts

Gallbladder

Cardinal point

Temporal bone

Cardiac plexus

Transverse colon

Hypogastric plexus

Pineal gland or epiphysis

Hypothalamus

Pituitary gland or hypophysis

Cardinal point   SBS

Tonsils and adenoids

Parathyroids

Thyroid

Thymus (T cells)

Heart

Cardiac plexus

Diaphragm

Duodenum

Gastroesophageal sphincter

Stomach

Pancreas

Solar plexus

Liver

Adrenal glands

Sensitive point for heart (on top of foot)

Kidneys

Pecquet's cistern

Duodenum

Sensitive point for the liver (on top of foot)

Ovaries or testicles

Bladder

Small intestine (ileum)

Small intestine (jejunum)

Ascending colon

Sigmoid colon

Rectum

Anus

Coccyx and cardinal point

Coccygeal plexus

Ischium and cardinal point

Cardinal point

Coronal or pineal plexus

Cardinal point

Hippocampus

Pituitary plexus

Thyroidal plexus

Lungs

Breasts

Cardinal point

Temporal bone

Spleen

Transverse colon

Descending colon

Hypogastric plexus

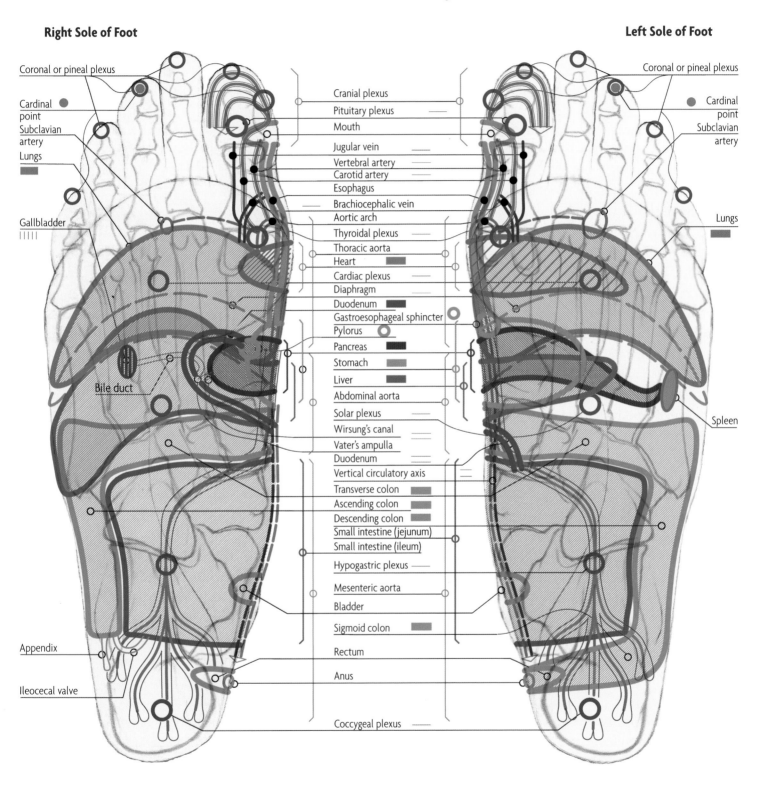

Right Sole of Foot

Left Sole of Foot

Coronal or pineal plexus

Cardinal point

Subclavian artery

Lungs

Gallbladder

Bile duct

Appendix

Ileocecal valve

Coronal or pineal plexus

Cardinal point

Subclavian artery

Lungs

Spleen

Cranial plexus
Pituitary plexus
Mouth
Jugular vein
Vertebral artery
Carotid artery
Esophagus
Brachiocephalic vein
Aortic arch
Thyroidal plexus
Thoracic aorta
Heart
Cardiac plexus
Diaphragm
Duodenum
Gastroesophageal sphincter
Pylorus
Pancreas
Stomach
Liver
Abdominal aorta
Solar plexus
Wirsung's canal
Vater's ampulla
Duodenum
Vertical circulatory axis
Transverse colon
Ascending colon
Descending colon
Small intestine (jejunum)
Small intestine (ileum)
Hypogastric plexus
Mesenteric aorta
Bladder
Sigmoid colon
Rectum
Anus
Coccygeal plexus

The Lymphatic System

A major part of the immune system, the lymphatic system is a complex network of lymph nodes, lymph ducts, lymphoid organs (bone marrow, spleen, and thymus), lymphatic tissues, lymph capillaries, and lymph vessels that produce lymph fluid and transport it from tissues to the circulatory system.

The lymphatic system has three interrelated functions: removal of excess fluids from the body tissues; absorption of fatty acids and subsequent transport of fat, as chyle, to the circulatory system; and production of immune cells such as lymphocytes (e.g., antibody-producing plasma cells) and monocytes.

The lymphatic vessels arise in the embryo from the veins, which they assist by aiding the circulation of fluid through large amounts of tissue. As the circular path through the body's system continues, the fluid is transported to progressively larger lymphatic vessels culminating in the right lymphatic duct (for lymph from the right upper body) and the thoracic duct (for the rest of the body); both ducts drain into the circulatory system at the right and left subclavian veins. The system collaborates with white blood cells in lymph nodes to protect the body from being infected by cancer cells, fungi, viruses, or bacteria. The brain, the spinal cord, bone marrow, and cartilage do not possess any lymphatic vessels or lymph nodes.

Unlike the vascular blood system, lymphatic circulation is dependent not upon the heart but upon the movement of the skeletal muscles of the arms and legs. Tight clothing can restrict movement of lymph, thus reducing the removal of wastes and allowing them to accumulate. If tissue fluid builds up, the tissue will swell; this is called edema. Clinical research in China has shown a 30 to 40 percent increase in the diameter of lymphatic venules and arterioles after a foot reflexology treatment. This increase optimizes the purifying function of lymph.

Before beginning a course of treatment, it is important to evaluate the state of the patient's immune system. One must also always keep in mind that the lymphatic vessels are the paths through which cancerous cells are distributed, or metastasized.

Because the immune system is based upon the balance of the liver, spleen, intestines, and autonomic nervous system, it is important to give these points particular focus during reflexology treatments.

Foot reflexology is effective for treating the immune system in cases of infections, circulatory problems, edemas, arthrosis or arthritis, and obesity (excess storage of fat). It also addresses immune functioning following trauma to the joints, in all states of stress, and during the aftereffects of surgery, especially mastectomy.

Locating the Reflex Zones of the Lymphatic System

The zone of the lymphatic system in the neck is in the "webbed" skin between the toes. The zone of the armpit lymphatic system is located over the head of the fifth metatarsal.

The zones of the abdomen's lymphatic system are located between the metatarsals and the heel on the sides of the feet. The zone for the cisterna chyli is located on the inner edge of the medial cuneiform bone. The zones for the pelvic lymphatic system are located on the heel, and the zones for the lymphatics of the groin are located on the top of the feet in an arc surrounding the ankle. The zones for the lymphatics of the breasts are on the top of the foot spanning the second through fifth metatarsals.

For an energy-based treatment of the lymphatic system, the reflexologist will focus on zone 1, which is connected to the vertebral column, and on the lymphatic glands of the intestines, as well as on zones 4 and 5 of the superficial lymph nodes. (See zone diagram on page 3.)

Right Sole of Foot

Left Sole of Foot

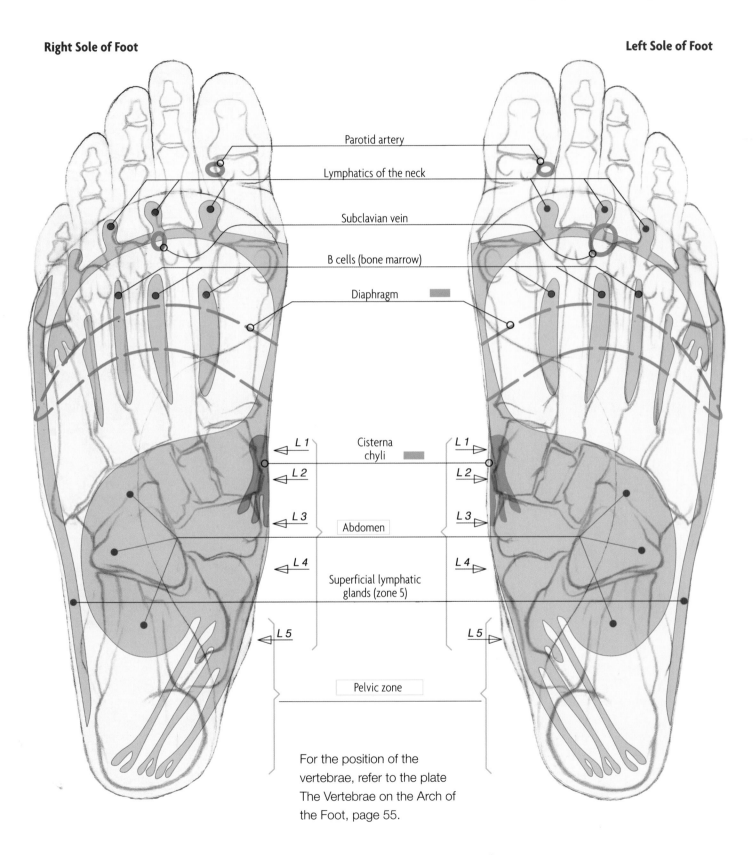

Parotid artery

Lymphatics of the neck

Subclavian vein

B cells (bone marrow)

Diaphragm

L 1   Cisterna   L 1
       chyli

L 2   L 2

L 3   Abdomen   L 3

L 4   Superficial lymphatic   L 4
       glands (zone 5)

L 5   L 5

Pelvic zone

For the position of the
vertebrae, refer to the plate
The Vertebrae on the Arch of
the Foot, page 55.

Left Top of Foot

Right Top of Foot

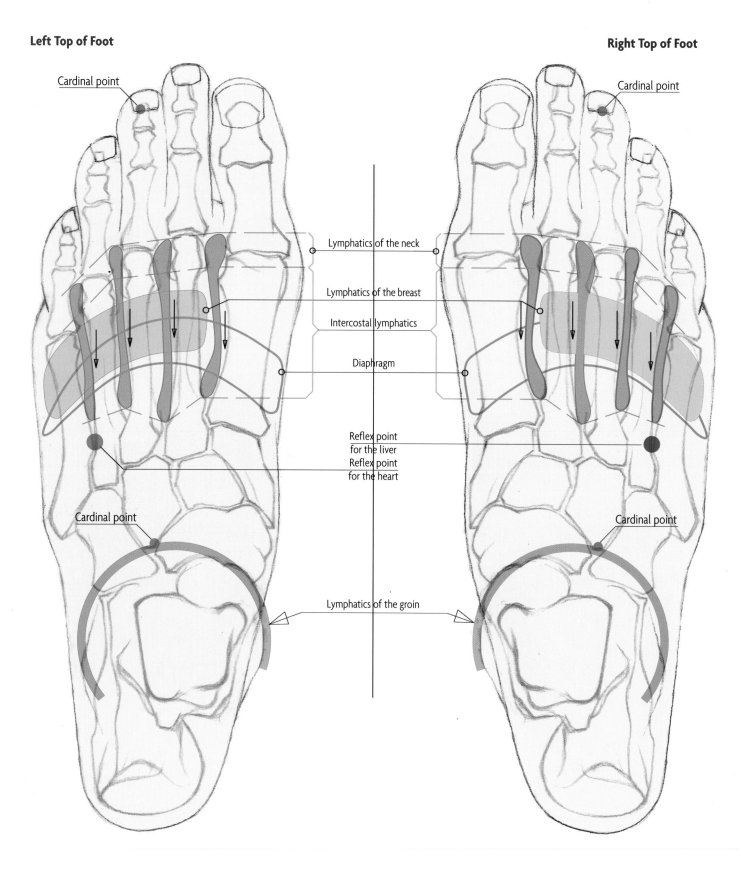

Cardinal point

Cardinal point

Lymphatics of the neck

Lymphatics of the breast

Intercostal lymphatics

Diaphragm

Reflex point
for the liver
Reflex point
for the heart

Cardinal point

Cardinal point

Lymphatics of the groin

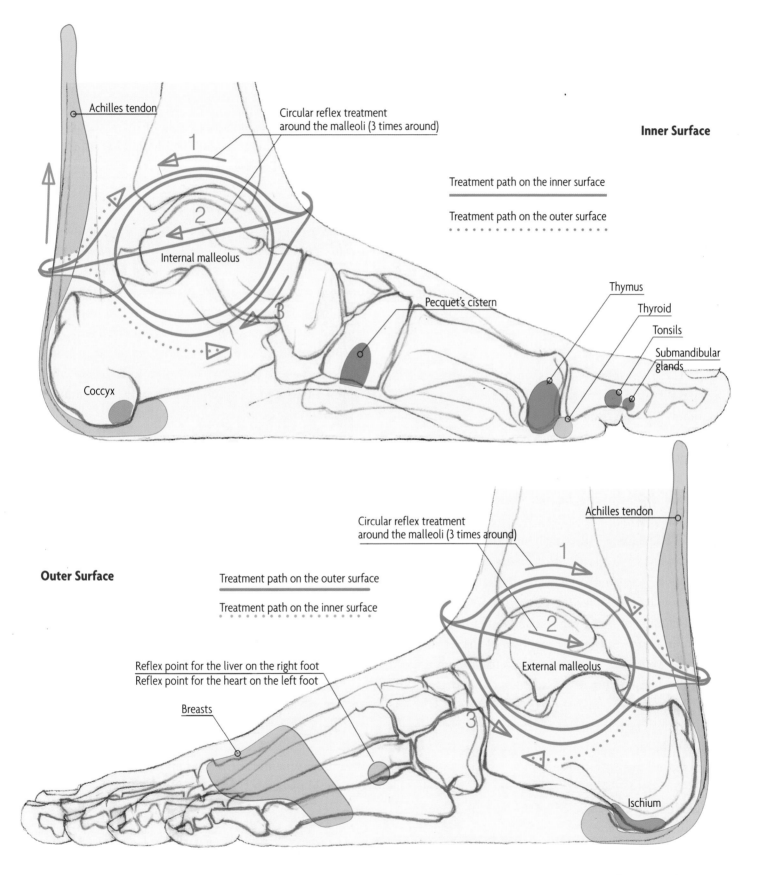

Inner Surface

Achilles tendon

Circular reflex treatment
around the malleoli (3 times around)

Treatment path on the inner surface

Treatment path on the outer surface

Internal malleolus

Pecquet's cistern

Thymus

Thyroid

Tonsils

Submandibular glands

Coccyx

Outer Surface

Treatment path on the outer surface

Treatment path on the inner surface

Circular reflex treatment
around the malleoli (3 times around)

Achilles tendon

External malleolus

Reflex point for the liver on the right foot
Reflex point for the heart on the left foot

Breasts

Ischium

Lymph

The fluid that flows through the lymphatic system is known as lymph. It is a clear, watery fluid derived from body tissues and contains white blood cells. Lymph acts to remove bacteria and certain proteins from the tissues, transport fat from the small intestine, and supply mature lymphocytes to the blood.

The lymphatic capillaries are tiny, thin-walled vessels that are closed at one end and are located in the spaces between cells throughout the body, except in the central nervous system and in nonvascular tissues. The main purpose of these vessels is to drain excess tissue fluids from around the cell ready to be filtered and returned to the venous circulation. Lymphatic capillaries are slightly larger in diameter than blood capillaries and have a unique structure that permits interstitial fluid to flow into them but not out. The lymphatic capillaries come together to form lymphatic vessels.

These vessels are divided into two plexuses: The superficial plexus meanders just below the skin and drains its lymph content into inguinal (inner thigh and groin), auxiliary (armpit), and cervical (head and neck) lymph nodes. The deep plexus is located in the thoracic and abdominal cavities and drains its lymph into the cisterna chyli, which is located along the vertebral column at level L2.

In addition to collecting lymph from the abdomen, the cisterna chyli receives proteins and lipids released by digestion. Reducing in size beneath the diaphragm, the cisterna chyli becomes the thoracic duct. The thoracic duct climbs up along the spinal column, to the left of the aorta, and ends at the junction of the left internal jugular vein and the subclavian vein. Already loaded with abdominal lymph, it also takes in lymph from the left lung, the legs, and the left side of the chest, neck, and head. The reflex point on the foot that corresponds to the thoracic duct is located between the big toe and the second toe.

The right lymphatic duct drains lymph from the right lung and the right side of the chest, neck, and head and terminates where the right internal jugular vein and right subclavian vein intersect.

It is through the lymphocytes that immune reactions develop in the lymph nodes (located on the paths of the lymphatic vessels).

Connective Tissue

Connective tissue plays a key role in the exchanges of the nervous, circulatory, and lymphatic systems and in the distribution of the CSF.

The Cerebrospinal Fluid

Located within the subarachnoid space of the meninges, the CSF plays an essential role in the immune system because of the antibodies it transports. It extends into the connective tissue, where it connects with the interstitial environment, the source zone for vein blood and lymph. The trauma of physical, emotional, mental, or spiritual whiplash can cause a blockage of the primary respiratory mechanism, which can in turn decrease the rate of the CSF's circulation and weaken the immune system and the body's resistance to disease.

Lymphocytes and Lymphoid Cells

During an infection, lymphocytes multiply in the lymphoid follicles and neutralize the infecting particles (antigens or immunogens). The thymus, which has a tendency to atrophy in the adult body, manufactures these lymphocytes. It plays a major role in the body's fight against infections and cancer.

The spleen, similar to the lymph nodes, filters the blood, recuperates the iron of red blood cells that are too old, stores lymphocytes, and, in certain metabolic disorders, stores large quantities of fat.

The tonsils, the adenoids, the ileocecal valve (the connection between the small and large intestines), and the appendix possess lymphoid tissue. Lymphoid follicles are also found in the liver and in the intestinal mucous membrane. This is known as gut-associated lymphoid tissue, or GALT.

Circulation of the Cerebrospinal Fluid

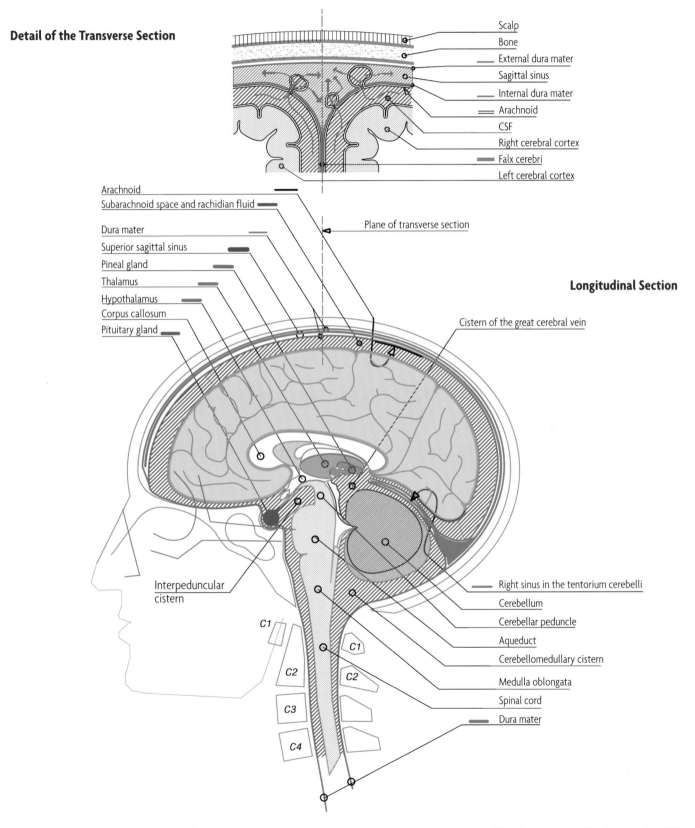

Detail of the Transverse Section

Scalp
Bone
External dura mater
Sagittal sinus
Internal dura mater
Arachnoid
CSF
Right cerebral cortex
Falx cerebri
Left cerebral cortex

Arachnoid
Subarachnoid space and rachidian fluid

Plane of transverse section

Dura mater
Superior sagittal sinus
Pineal gland
Thalamus
Hypothalamus
Corpus callosum
Pituitary gland

Longitudinal Section

Cistern of the great cerebral vein

Interpeduncular cistern

C1
C2
C3
C4

C1
C2

Right sinus in the tentorium cerebelli
Cerebellum
Cerebellar peduncle
Aqueduct
Cerebellomedullary cistern
Medulla oblongata
Spinal cord
Dura mater

The Immune System

The immune system varies in its effectiveness according to age, sex, genetic factors, and nutrition. A natural immune system is present in the infant, but his or her acquired immunity to specific diseases comes from the antibodies provided by the mother during the first six months of nursing. Lymphocytes mature at a slower rate as we get older, so the immune defenses of elderly people are much weaker than those of their younger counterparts. Before menopause, women have much more effective immune systems than men thanks to their very active hormonal systems.

Deficiencies in zinc and vitamins C and B, along with excessive consumption of animal proteins, weaken the natural immune system.

Fever and inflammation have a beneficial effect on the natural immune system because they increase the migration of macrophages, stimulating antiviral activity. Natural therapies, instead of bringing these symptoms to an abrupt halt, respect their vital evolution while guiding their effects for the patient's benefit.

A deficient genetic makeup or a poor diet weakens the body's natural immune system, as do stress and emotional traumas, which stimulate the adrenal-hypthalamo-pituitary axis. Producing an excess of adrenaline, glucagons, and cortisol, this axis has an anti-inflammatory effect but also increases blood sugar levels and raises blood pressure. It is important to keep this process in mind when treating patients suffering from chronic illness or those dealing with longstanding and recurring stressors.

The skin, which forms a barrier, and sweat, whose moderate acidity protects the digestive, nasopharyngeal, and urogenital membranes, together make up the immune system's first line of defense. The body also produces natural antibiotics (phagocytes) and natural antiviral cells (interferons).

Acquired immunity operates through lymphocytes that are specific to every kind of previously encountered antigen. Once an antigen has been identified for the first time, its identity is held in the body's memory and it is henceforth recognized by the body. When a previously defeated antigen makes a new appearance, the immune system's reaction will be much faster and much more intense. (This is the principle behind vaccination.)

B cells circulating in the blood serum, the interstitial fluid, lymph, saliva, and vaginal secretions also provide antibodies for neutralizing antigens.

When the body is confronted with specific, particularly aggressive antigens, T cells pick up the relay of the immune system's defenses. Produced in the thymus, they do not secrete antibodies but recognize what is of the "self"; this is called the human leukocyte antigen (HLA) system. The T cells then activate macrophages or destroy the cells infected by the virus themselves, thereby protecting the cells that have not yet been affected.

If these T cells no longer recognize the HLA system, they then attack the healthy cells they are responsible for protecting. This phenomenon is at play in autoimmune diseases such as lupus, polyarthritis, spondylarthritis, psoriasis, multiple sclerosis, Basedow's disease, allergy-induced asthma, and so on.

The immune system relies on the balanced function of the liver, the spleen, the intestines, and the autonomic nervous system. When a profound stress has not been fully integrated, the body falls into a sympathicotonic state that brings with it a constant release of adrenaline, which then causes symptoms such as sleep disorders, fatigue, weight loss, and poor digestion. This has an echo effect upon the entire glandular system of the body, with the immune system most strongly affected.

The irritable or depressed mood brought about by stress can create one of two responses: either the subject becomes conscious of what is happening, thus allowing the body to enter a parasympathicotonic state, or the warning signal is not perceived and the individual forces his or her body to keep going, with an increasing reliance on stimulants such as coffee, tobacco, alcohol, psychotropic drugs, and so on.

Whereas becoming conscious of stress brings about a positive attitude and consequently a physical reaction that maximizes immune function, conversely, ignoring stress creates a negative attitude and leaves the body

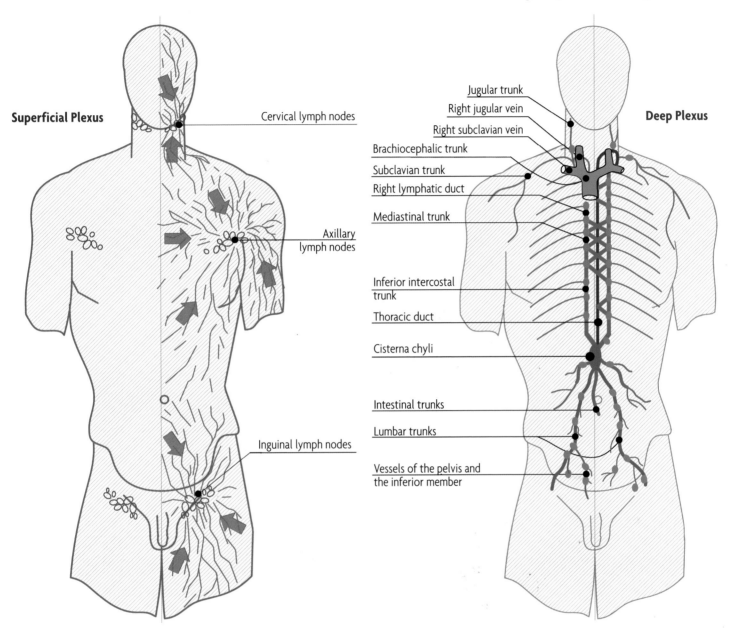

Superficial Plexus

Cervical lymph nodes

Axillary
lymph nodes

Inguinal lymph nodes

Jugular trunk
Right jugular vein
Right subclavian vein
Brachiocephalic trunk
Subclavian trunk
Right lymphatic duct
Mediastinal trunk

Inferior intercostal
trunk
Thoracic duct
Cisterna chyli

Intestinal trunks
Lumbar trunks

Vessels of the pelvis and
the inferior member

Deep Plexus

more vulnerable. The immune system grows weaker, and the least virus or bacterium (innocuous under regular circumstances) can wreak havoc. It's as if the consciousness that inhabits the body, giving it life, has taken leave, so the outer form begins to deteriorate.

Our bodies are home to millions of viruses, bacteria, and funguses. They're part of life, contributing to the body's ongoing quest for balance. This interac-

tion is felt most keenly when a state of mental fragility exists or when an organ is depleted of energy. The body can then invite one of its bacterial or viral guests to take part in the healing process and the reorganization of the body through some clearing (discharge of pus or other substances). This elimination requires heat and increased body temperature, as well as rest and time to reflect.

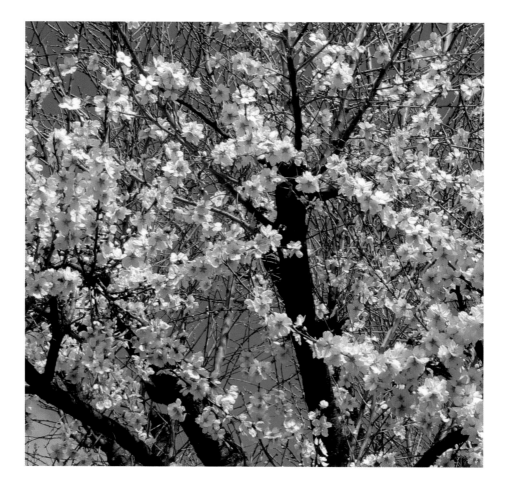

PART FOUR

A Healthy Lifestyle

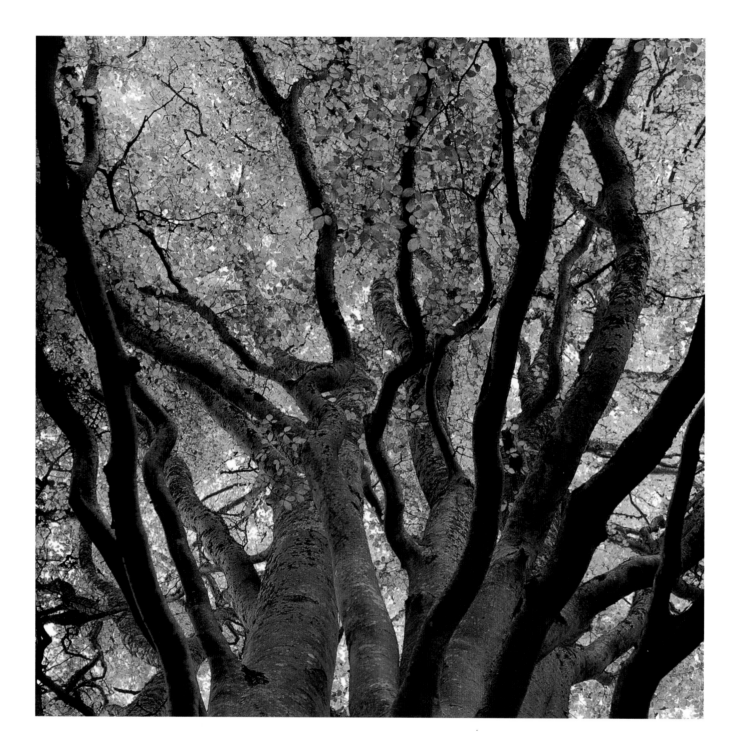

The Vital Force

Every being possesses an intelligent vital force that preserves and maintains the spiritual, psychic, and material cohesion of the cells of which it is made. This force is life itself; it is the badge of the spirit, the internal doctor, intuition, and common sense.

The vital force is subject to the influences of the environment even as it adapts to them. It animates mental life, physical life, and emotional life. It is the source of thought and creativity and gives life to inspiration.

When the body suffers from a strong emotion, a shock, a stress, or a virus, the first to be disturbed is its vital force. It responds with some electromagnetic modification that stimulates the body's defense mechanism, sets the autonomic nervous system in motion, and sets off chain reactions in the physical, emotional, or mental realm. When disease emerges, its very first stage involves a defensive reaction that is metabolic in nature. This reaction is a manifestation of the vital force.

Therapies that harness the vital force, such as acupuncture, homeopathy, phytotherapy, and reflexology, act directly—slowly but thoroughly—on the stress or illness causing disruption. These therapies are the instruments, but only the vital force actually does the healing. It is the vital force that determines what the body's priorities are with respect to the needs of the patient.

In all natural therapies, but particularly in reflexology, the patient's basic vital force should be evaluated with the greatest attention. The frequency and intensity of the treatment to follow will depend upon this initial diagnosis.

The activity performed by the vital force is quite diverse in nature. To protect the body, depending on what elements are deficient, it transforms minerals in the following ways: potassium into sodium, magnesium into calcium, iron into manganese, and silica into aluminum. It preserves the dynamic balance of the body, from its form and structure down to its cellular constitution. Every living being is constantly receiving and emitting energy in the form of radiation, thoughts, or feelings, which all have a bearing on its equilibrium.

Reception and Emission

The perpetual interplay between these two dynamics, reception and emission, forms the very principle of life. Centrifugal force opens us to all that calls our attention from the outside, whether positive or negative. Centripetal force pulls us back within ourselves. Form exists only as the result of the balance of these two forces.

If there is an excess of incoming energy, rigidification and sclerosis, then crystallization, will result in the body's tissues. Personality also comes into play here. In the case of inhibition and excess incoming energy, for example, the body will put up a resistance that will inhibit metabolism.

Any emission of energy comes from the release of heat, along with the dissolution of physical or psychic cohesion. This applies to fever, a hot abscess with the elimination of pus, or even an emotional outburst accompanied by flushed cheeks and a torrent of words. Here, too, personality is an important factor, as it is crucial to be able to express oneself.

A person's constitution may dictate which dynamic predominates. Each tendency goes with certain aspects of the personality and even physical structure.

Centripetal Tendency

Positive aspects: This person will be precise and efficient. Centripetal movement and the maintenance of structure rely on mental activity.

Negative aspects: Plans and ideas for the centripetal type tend to be rigid and hard-edged. The personality is cold, overly structured, depressive, and introverted. Sclerosis is a frequent physical result. Communication is restrained.

Centrifugal Tendency

Positive aspects: This personality is extroverted, warm, and open to communication. The individual has a strong need to be in relationship with other forms of life. Centrifugal movement and radiation of energy affect emotional life.

Negative aspects: Centrifugal tendency generates excessive activity. The person may be overly talkative, with a great deal of gesticulating. He or she may lack control and self-restraint.

Either dynamic may predominate temporarily based on circumstances. The two phases can even alternate in the same individual.

In order to adapt to the constant modifications of its environment while preserving its structure, the human body has established a system of biofeedback or self-regulation. This mechanism ensures the maintenance of the body's structure and the fulfillment of its functions.

All self-regulation consists of three successive stages:

Reception: The receptors are characterized by their sensitivity to specific types of energy: chemical, luminous, vibratory, and mechanical.

Transmission: The stimulation of a receptor triggers a chemical alarm bell through the production and expulsion of a specific substance—the transmitter, or the mediator. The transmitter influences the cells in the immediate proximity of its site of emission (primary mediator), then it is transported a great distance by the bloodstream as well as the circulatory networks of the nervous, lymphatic, hormonal, and energetic systems to its needed location.

Action: The action varies depending upon the nature of the mediators and the targeted areas (the effectors). The effectors in response to the mediators perform some chemical or mechanical task. The muscular tissues, for example, are mechanical effectors.

Reflexology has the role of harmonizing this self-regulating energetic circulation. It achieves this by interfacing with all the emotional and mental aspects of the being. As mentioned earlier, the reflexologist should, as a preliminary step, evaluate the overall vital force of the patient and that of the precise organ or zone being treated. The practitioner's listening skills and ability to pay attention are crucial to taking into consideration all aspects of a patient's history.

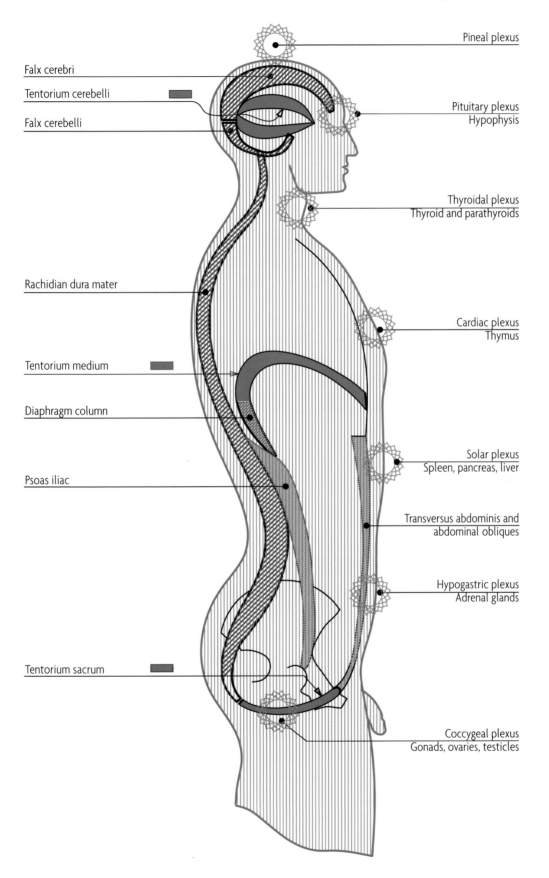

Pineal plexus

Falx cerebri

Tentorium cerebelli

Falx cerebelli

Pituitary plexus
Hypophysis

Thyroidal plexus
Thyroid and parathyroids

Rachidian dura mater

Cardiac plexus
Thymus

Tentorium medium

Diaphragm column

Solar plexus
Spleen, pancreas, liver

Psoas iliac

Transversus abdominis and
abdominal obliques

Hypogastric plexus
Adrenal glands

Tentorium sacrum

Coccygeal plexus
Gonads, ovaries, testicles

The Forces of Life

Where does the body begin and where does it end? At what distance from the skin can one still interact with the body's energetic field? This field, which we can interpret as a mysterious life force, gives birth to the electromagnetic radiations that diminish proportionately to their distance from their radiant source—but they never cease to radiate, just like other fields that propagate throughout the universe.

In alternative and natural therapies, energy is the force that alters the patient's vital force. The beating of the heart, the movement of the legs, muscles, and tendons—all use chemical energy converted into mechanical energy. The latter is stored as potential energy in the muscles and tendons of the body.

A cell is a sac containing chemical substances gathered together in a cytoplasmic solution where biochemical reactions take place. These cells also contain fibers, tubes, and filaments that cross the cytoplasmic matrix and link the interior to the exterior. Known as "integrins," these cells unite the nucleolar matter with the surrounding connective tissues. This creates the system that allows information, by means of chemical transformations, to be conveyed from the genes to the connective tissues to the skin.

By treating the sole of the foot, the reflexologist mobilizes the external energy of the skin and transfers it, via the reflex arc, from the tissue to the cell nucleus, which will memorize the information that passes through it.

Electromagnetic Energy in the Body

The body produces an electric current and a magnetic current that interact with each other. The different tissues of the body generate a multitude of electromagnetic fields. The strongest of these fields is that created by the heart and its large vessels; it can be measured from a distance of six yards. Composed of numerous ions and charged by magnetic electrons (minerals, iron in particular), blood is an excellent conductor of electricity. The heartbeat sends blood pulsing through all the cavities of the body and through its large vessels in a spiral movement, creating a pulsing and harmonious magnetic field.

Experiments performed in 1990 demonstrated that the hands of the therapist emit strong magnetic impulses that join with the biomagnetic field of the patient. According to quantum theory, when two waves meet, they will combine to create a magnetic field whose sum is greater than the whole of its parts and carries a wealth of information.

The tissues, cells, molecules, and atoms—the elementary particles of the body—formulate a secret language whose meaning we are just beginning to grasp. The aura or magnetic field could be understood as the manifestation of the sum total of all the body's energies. Every part of the body is in direct and constant contact with all the other parts. Is this chemical, mechanical, electrical, and electromagnetic communication what energy is? At the very least, it is what forms the principle of holism or homeostasis.

Every day, 98 percent of the body's atoms are renewed. How do the cells know when it is time for them to be replaced? How is the integrity of the body's structure preserved during this constant process of renewal? It is plausible that there is a vital force that protects all the elements of the body in the interest of the continuity of life and the perpetuation of the species.

The Chakras

The Plexuses

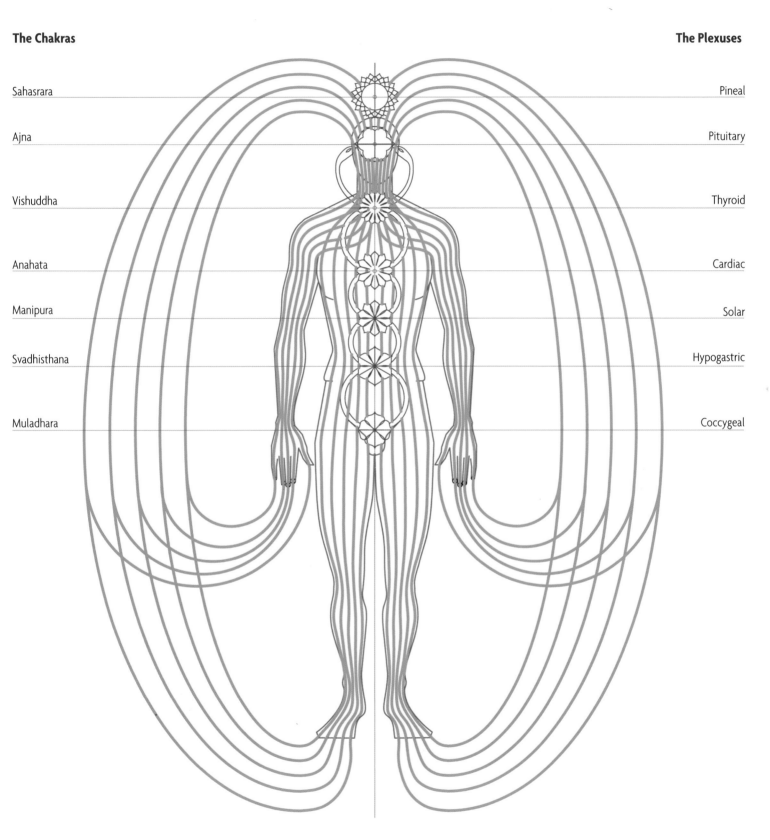

Sahasrara — Pineal

Ajna — Pituitary

Vishuddha — Thyroid

Anahata — Cardiac

Manipura — Solar

Svadhisthana — Hypogastric

Muladhara — Coccygeal

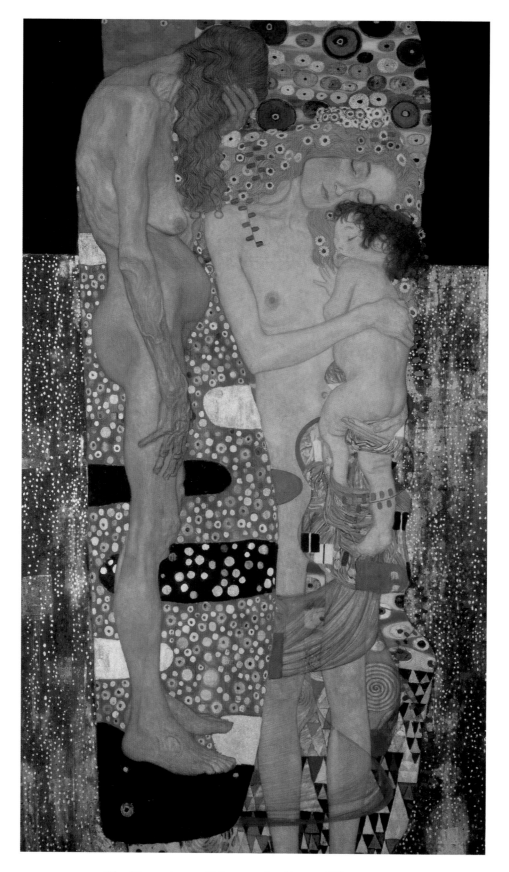

The Three Ages of Woman, *by Gustav Klimt, Rome,*
Galleria Nazionale d'arte Moderna e Contemporanea

The Phenomenon of Aging

Life expectancy increases every year now. Treating physical deterioration due to age is becoming as common for therapists as treating disease.

Aging begins in the brain. Research on Alzheimer's disease has brought to light certain mechanisms of cerebral aging—in particular, that of memory.

Memory and Cerebral Zone

Neuroimaging has made it possible to precisely pinpoint the zones of the brain that are involved in the different forms of memory. In the cerebral cortex, the temporal lobe is the seat of long-term memory, and the putamen is the seat of functional memory, where acquired behavior (riding a bicycle, for example) is located.

In the limbic brain, there are three parts associated with memory. The hippocampus is the memory bank. The amygdala is the seat of unconscious memory and guarantees the relay of emotional memories; it stores away traumatic episodes. The caudate nucleus is the seat of instinct, genetic memory, and the coded memory of the past.

Different zones of the brain are activated simultaneously when a piece of information is encoded or recalled. Memories and newly acquired information are stored through various networks of different zones; they are recalled to govern behavior.

Forgotten from Memory

The brain internalizes the outside world. Using signals provided by the environment, it constructs representations that are no longer just a simple reflection of reality. These representations guide our actions. Each one has a corresponding temporary network of neurons.

Years after a concert, a melody will float back into memory. This melody has left an imprint, or amnesic trace. Cells and neurons within the hippocampus that were initially deaf respond when this sound is heard. The trace of the memory is inscribed in the synapses, where it can be evoked by this sound. Years after it was "learned," this sound can reappear in the mind.

Inactive memory is a latent or potential form of remembering in which the altered synapses guide access to the sleeping memory. It could be said that memory is a psychological concept, an organized collection of representations of events and the relationships among them. Synaptic plasticity (the ability of the synapses to change) is, on the other hand, a neurobiological concept.

Forgetting goes hand in hand with the disappearance of the synaptic modifications connected with the "learning" of something once remembered. But is the forgetting absolute? It is not known whether a "forgotten" memory has actually been erased or if it has simply become inaccessible.

The Causes of Cerebral Aging

There are several physiological factors that need to be taken into account in the aging process:

▶ Certain changes in cognitive capacities (reduction of visual acuity, hearing loss, diminishment of the sense of taste or of touch, increased imbalance) lead the subject to feel increasingly isolated.

▶ A reduction in the consumption of glucose and oxygen occurs in the temporal lobe, where the structures responsible for the formation of memories and the learning of language are housed (the hippocampus and the amygdala). This reduction alters synaptic activity and neurotransmission. There is also a drop in the levels of noradrenaline, serotonin, and dopamine.

- Morphological modifications take place, including cortical atrophy accompanied by a dilation of the cerebral ventricles and neuronal loss.
- Genetic mutations will cause changes in the chromosomes of the cells' nuclei.
- Inactivity of the thymus causes reduced immunity; slowdown of the pituitary gland causes decreased endocrine secretions.

Certain external factors also contribute to senescence:

- Free radicals—toxic oxidizing molecules produced by the body following assaults from the environment—affect cellular membranes and genetic material.
- Toxic substances like lead, steel, mercury, and aluminum cause some deterioration of neurons.
- Stress, with its oxidizing effect, also takes a toll.

Certain sociocultural factors also come into play. Western societies do not value old age, which they associate with dependence, incompetence, and senility. Once isolated in this way, the aged individual loses all initiative. His or her individual experience, which has been inscribed in the brain permanently in the connections among neurons, becomes impoverished.

Synaptic efficiency relies on the activity of the neurons located throughout the synapse. This functional cerebral plasticity is the result of neurobiological and environmental interactions, so a decrease in these interactions (isolation and boredom) leads to decreased neuronal activity and results in lower synaptic efficiency.

Cellular aging begins in the septum pellucidum, located within the hippocampus, and in the temporal lobe. In these two zones are the nervous cells that are the most vulnerable to ischemia, which causes memory problems after or during a traumatic event. Furthermore, it has been observed that if the functioning of the hippocampus is impeded, there is a loss of spatial memory.

Cerebral aging is measured by the reduction of the brain's weight, neuronal loss, neurofibrillary deterioration, senile plaques, and a change in cholinergic function, resulting in cognitive difficulties.

Preventive Measures

Neuronal Gymnastics

Despite all of these various factors, cerebral plasticity makes it possible to maintain cognitive capabilities and to support intellectual activities because the neurons retain the ability to remodel their circuits, to alter already existing synaptic connections, and even to forge new ones.

Intellectual gymnastics and creativity are the best means of stimulating the neurons. Intellectual exercise can compensate for the decline of cognitive faculties because, while the gray matter has a tendency to shrink in volume and weight, the richness of conceiving and developing creative projects has positive effects on memory function. Useful intellectual exercises include reciting texts, memorizing verse, and playing chess, as well as teaching and passing on one's knowledge in various ways.

Diet

Foods containing antioxidants play an essential role here. The body eliminates free radicals through the action of selenium, zinc, and certain vitamins (E, C, and A).

Breathing

Oxygen and glucose guarantee the functioning and survival of neurons thanks to the blood, which is the primary transporter of fuel. This is why deep breathing is so important, as is physical exercise that requires the use of numerous mental capabilities (concentration, attention, memorization). This has beneficial effects both on the body in general and on the brain in particular.

Aging Well

While all of us age, we do not all grow old in the same fashion. Successful aging is a consequence of lifestyle, habits, and psychosocial factors. The state of youth is that of holding energy. Its very essence is evolution toward more and better. Aging, on the other hand, is exhibited by an involution, a change toward less: there is loss of energy, loss of trust in life, loss of the sensory tools for communication. The elderly no longer hear, no longer look, and no longer see—even before losing their eyesight. They no longer work, then no longer play, and finally lose all love of life.

In order to resist aging, it is necessary to exercise all of one's faculties. To continue living as fully as possible is to know how to age, for accepting the fact of old age is part of managing the fear of death.

The Effect of Reflexology on Aging

Reflexology makes it possible to slow the aging process and to keep the organs and senses functioning well. These functions are often altered during senescence with the loss of memory, sensation, and motivation and the loss of analytical faculties and coordination. Reflex massage improves and stimulates cellular renewal. The stimulation of all sectors of a given zone can have a profound impact on other zones at a distance (for example, a blocked zone on the foot often affects the occipital zones of vision in the brain).

In order to use reflexology in the most effective way, there are a number of fundamental facts and principles to remember.

1. The key points to work on the foot for the circulation of the brain are:
   * The ten zones reproduced on the two big toes. (See page 136.) These demand particular attention, especially on the upper, lower, and lateral parts.
   * The cerebral zones (hippocampus, limbic brain, pituitary gland, pineal gland, carotid and vertebral arteries). These should be treated millimeter by millimeter in order to stimulate every cell of the brain and activate blood, lymph, and CSF circulation.
   * The joint between P1 and P2 of the big toe—on its lower part, around the foramen magnum and the occipital condyles where the atlas hooks onto the occiput, and on its upper part, on the bones of the cranial vault and their occipital, temporal, sphenoidal, and frontal sutures. (See page 55.)
2. The twelve pairs of cranial nerves should be treated carefully on each of the four toes, as aging first affects the organs of the senses—ears, eyes, nose, tongue, and skin. (See page 127.)

3. The reflexology treatment of the craniosacral system covers all the zones. This treatment should be performed by working on the reflex points for both parts, the skull and the sacrum, as well as on the points for the spinal column and the rachidian nerves.
4. The stimulation of the point for a single hormonal gland on the foot impacts all the others. It is therefore quite important to fully grasp the extent of their interactions and not to undertake a fragmented treatment of symptoms.

To Slow Down the Aging Process

▶ Live without regrets and with a calm and peaceful heart.
▶ Cultivate optimism and an open mind.
▶ Be happy in spirit, and remain calm and tranquil.
▶ Learn how to laugh at yourself.
▶ Cultivate the simple wisdom of everyday life.
▶ Learn how to listen to your body and its needs. It will reward you with well-being.
▶ Avoid both anger and frustration.
▶ Avoid anxiety and dwelling on problems.
▶ Exercise without going to extremes, preferably outdoors. Walking and calisthenics are recommended even until very late in life. Better to do these in the morning than the evening.
▶ Establish and respect the rhythms of daily habits (getting up, grooming, dressing, regular mealtimes).
▶ Avoid tobacco and drinking alcohol in excess (no more than one glass of wine per meal).
▶ Eat moderately. Drink green tea and lots of water.
▶ Cultivate hobbies: games, chess, cards, calligraphy, painting, music, gardening, fishing, and so on. This will increase one's zest for living.
▶ A serene spirit and wise mind pair naturally with health and energy.

We can be old at any age—youth is simply a state of mind. The more we exercise our abilities, the better we resist old age. Over the generations, we've grown old later and later in life.

In short: die young . . . but as late as possible!

When You Are Very Old

When you are very old, one evening by candlelight,
seated by the fire, spooling and spinning,
you will tell yourself, while singing my verses in amazement:
"Ronsard celebrated me when I was fair."
Then not a one of your servants gently dozing there,
lulled by your labor, will at the sound of my name
start from her slumbers
and bless your name with immortal praise.

I will be beneath the ground a boneless phantom
taking my long rest beneath the myrtle shade,
while you are an old woman stooped before the hearth,
regretting my love and your haughty disdain.
Heed what I say and live for today, await not tomorrow.
Pluck today the roses of life.

Sonnets for Hélène, Pierre de Ronsard

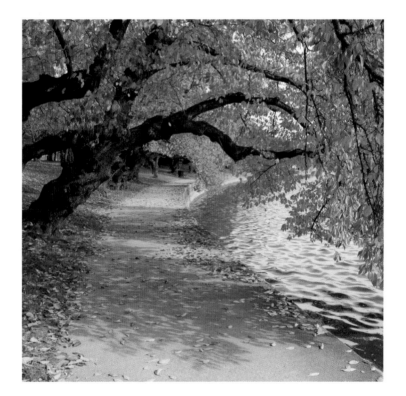

Autumn

WHEN YOU WANT TO FIND A GIRLFRIEND

Take her in the beauty of age
When her mind is fully awakened
And her breasts are nicely rounded
A tender
Heart
Most sensible
In language
Dancing, singing in fine harmony
And firm in heart and body.

If you take her too young
You will not understand one another.
For lasting relationship take the brunette
A brownie point for ensuring its support
One good turn
Deserves another
When one goes
On hunt
For the pleasant game of love
The one who captures such prey is happy.

CLÉMENT MAROT, *CHANSONS*

Advice for Living Well

According to Hubert Reeves, joy and the pleasures offered by life are essential for us to bloom and cultivate an open mind and positive thinking. Our thoughts and emotions act on our physical, mental, and psychological health, as these three aspects are inseparable.

Biorhythms

To live to a ripe old age and enjoy good health, it is necessary to understand how biorhythms—reflections of the different annual, seasonal, monthly, and daily cycles—influence "chi," or energy. Spring is the time of the renewal of nature. This yang period lasts until the end of summer, when it makes way for the yin period of fall and winter.

The body, too, has its rhythms: for example, it is better to exercise in the morning with the rising sun, which is yang, and not during the evening when the sun is setting, a yin period of the day. Harmony is found between yin and yang. Those who live drawing too strongly from one of these poles at the expense of the other exhaust their energy. Yin deficiencies are responsible for the symptoms that are most commonly found in our modern societies.

To start the day on the right foot, implement the following habits: Rise with the sun, perform abdominal exercises, and take deep breaths; when washing in the morning, end with cold water; take a walk in the fresh air, taking time to admire the trees and all the beauty of nature; eat breakfast in a tranquil environment; rest for several minutes before leaving for work.

To keep the day going well, take a rest around noon (the ideal siesta is between 11:00 AM and 1:00 PM) and adopt a healthy diet.

And to bring each day to a good close, avoid eating the evening meal too late, and eat modest amounts of food, avoiding alcohol. Go to bed around 10:00 PM (and no later than 11:00 PM). Get plenty of sleep.

The Art of Breathing

Every morning and evening, you should practice abdominal breathing. To do this, take a very deep breath, and when exhaling, pay special attention to the lower abdomen to make sure all air is pushed out, with the mouth open and the eyes closed. Breathe this way several times, slowly and with concentration.

Water Is the Best Medicine

Water is the principal constituent of the human body and the key element involved in the process of absorption and evaporation: we take it in through drink and the ambient humidity, then release it through respiration, transpiration, and urinary evacuation. Rainwater, which is naturally soft, is the best. Tap water, which is much harder, contains oxides. It should be softened and purified with filters; these will remove the nitrates that come from fertilizers, chlorides, and chemical toxins.

Drinking a cup of boiled water, still hot, each morning will encourage the action of yang. Generally speaking, one should drink warm beverages when the body is cold. Ice water counters the effects of alcohol and lowers the body's temperature in the case of fever, but otherwise, it is not advised to drink water that cold.

To maintain the quantity and quality of the body's water, develop the following habits:

▶ Maintain tranquillity and peace of mind.

- ▶ Take a nap at the beginning of the afternoon.
- ▶ Learn to relax.
- ▶ Breathe regularly through the abdomen.
- ▶ Keep your mouth closed.
- ▶ Sleep on your side.
- ▶ Exercise in the morning, before the day's temperatures have climbed too high, in order to avoid perspiring heavily.
- ▶ Drink water frequently in small amounts at a time; make sure that it is of good quality and drink two to three liters total a day.
- ▶ Eat foods that are not too dry.
- ▶ To increase the production of saliva, chew your food more. You may also want to practice the following exercise: Close your mouth and clamp your teeth together for several seconds.

For more information on the importance of water, see the chapter The Healing Power of Water.

Grooming and Hygiene

Washing oneself is an art that contributes to relaxation. Daily ablutions clean out the pores, stimulate blood circulation, and regulate the different energies of the body.

In the morning, wash your face with cold water or take a cold shower: cold water not only stimulates the circulatory system and the nervous system but also activates the immune system.

A warm bath should not be taken in the morning because it will carry energy to the surface of the skin, thus taking yang from the rest of the body. A reasonably warm bath may be taken in the evening before going to bed.

Saunas are not recommended for those in poor health or for pregnant, lactating, or menstruating women. However, saunas do increase energy for people in good health.

Getting fresh air, bathing in seawater, sunbathing in the morning, and taking walks in the woods—all help regulate the body's energies. This happens simply through relaxation and improved circulation.

Eating Correctly

Eat a large breakfast, a medium-sized lunch, and a light dinner. Keep negative emotions away from the table. Arguments and the settling of scores should happen elsewhere. Avoid alcohol, stimulants, unnatural additives and substitutes, and unhealthy food combinations.

Eat lightly, as slowly and as healthily as possible, allowing four or five hours between each meal. To stop hunger pangs between meals, drink a glass of water. Fruits should be eaten before meals.

Good Elimination

The chimneys and pipes must be in perfect order for a house to function well. The same holds true for the body with respect to clearing out nasal mucus, abdominal and stomach gases, and feces; all must be evacuated regularly to avoid any kind of stasis. As "death begins in the intestines," all steps should be taken to maintain good intestinal transit. Stress, nervous tension, lack of water, and foods that are either too rich or too dry are all detrimental to good elimination. Equally detrimental in this regard is an egotistical mentality.

Sexual Energy

A sexual exchange between a man and a woman (yang and yin) can have the result of prolonging life and, even better, helping the body fight off illness. However, there are certain rules that should be observed:

Sexual desire is still a part of life in old age. There is wisdom in knowing how to keep health and happiness in this vital activity. Extreme abstinence will bring about frustration and resentment and destroy the equilibrium between the two partners.

Remember that the quality of the act is just as important as the frequency with which it occurs. Mutual exchange, love, and satisfaction are the important things to focus on. Fatigue and sorrow following the sexual act are signs of a problem.

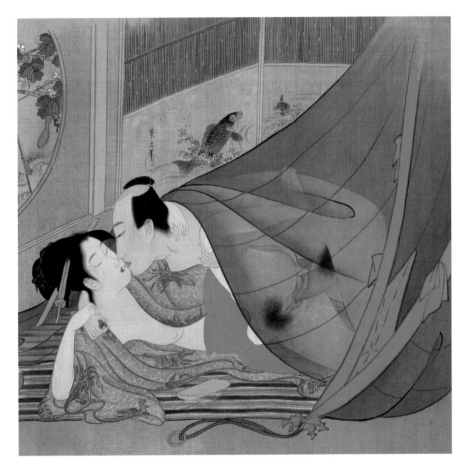

Image from The Floating World, *Japan*

Sleep

A human being spends a third of his or her life sleeping, but this recuperative time varies in length from one person to the next. There are some people who feel just fine with four or five hours of sleep, whereas others need ten hours. The quality of one's sleep is of fundamental importance.

Sleep research has shown that the first ninety minutes are what's known as "deep sleep," followed by the period during which the brain waves (alpha waves) slow down; it is very difficult to wake up during this time. Next comes the rapid eye movement (REM) phase, which is accompanied by an acceleration of the heartbeat. This is the period of dreaming. It constitutes one-fourth of sleep time and alternates with periods of slow waves. Awakening occurs at the end of a REM period.

Brain activity, which is quite intense during sleep, is vital for health. Research has shown that during the alpha-wave sleep phase, the pituitary gland secretes growth hormones and the metabolism of fats and proteins, essential for the repair of the body's tissues, becomes very active. The rapid-wave phase (REM) acts upon the central nervous system's entire network of circuits. This is also when the pineal gland synthesizes melatonin to stimulate the thyroid, the adrenal glands, and the sexual glands.

Restorative sleep is characterized by its rapid onset and slow and rhythmic breathing; there should be no snoring, nightmares, or waking up during the night. In the morning, the mind should feel clear and serene; and the body, rested.

Alcohol, caffeine, and other drugs disturb the cerebral rhythm of sleep. A disrupted REM period can cause a lack of concentration, memory trouble, and an inability to learn. The two hours before midnight are the most beneficial for resting because they coincide with the first slow waves of the body's deep restoration period.

In order to get a good night's sleep, respect the following principles:

▶ During the day, avoid pushing yourself beyond your limits, both intellectually and physically, particularly between 5:00 and 7:00 PM.
▶ Take a nap for at least twenty minutes.
▶ Don't forget that alcohol and caffeine are stimulants, as are television and movies.
▶ Save any worries that show up at night for the yang period of the morning. Their solution will be easier to find then.
▶ The evening meal shouldn't start too late and the food shouldn't be too hot; take your time eating.
▶ Make sure your feet are warm before you go to bed.
▶ Prepare your mind for sleep with meditation; the body will follow right after.
▶ Your bedroom should be well ventilated and neither too hot, too cold, nor too dry.
▶ You should sleep with your head pointing to the north.
▶ Keep your mouth closed to avoid dehydration.
▶ Go to sleep lying on your right side.

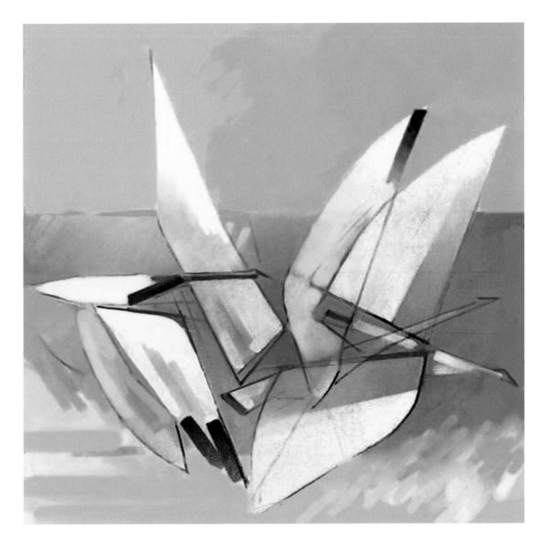

Flight

The Brain of the Heart

During the earliest heart transplants, it was discovered—and this was a source of great surprise—that the heart is the privileged site for emotion. Physiology as taught at the time maintained that the heart was a simple pump: it could be unclogged through stent procedures; parts of its piping could be replaced with bypass surgery; and when the damage was too far gone, the whole thing could be replaced. This completely discounted the folk wisdom that has always seen the heart as the seat of tenderness, love, courage, and generosity.

Biologically speaking, the heart is a remarkably efficient organ. It works nonstop, sometimes for more than ninety years, at a rhythm of 100,000 beats per day, pumping around eight liters of blood per minute during normal activity and around five liters when the body is at rest through a vascular system that is 60,000 miles long (more than twice the circumference of the earth). Among the magnetic fields that the body produces, the heart's is the most powerful. It surrounds the body and even extends some distance beyond it.

Even before the brain has formed, the heart is beating in the fetus. It is not even known what triggers its pulsations; their source seems to lie within the heart itself. It is believed that the central nervous system controls them; however, the heart has no need of the brain to do its work: during a transplant, the nerves connecting heart to brain are severed, but the heart keeps beating.

The Intelligence of the Heart

During the 1970s, the Laceys, a couple who were American physiologists, discovered that the heart has an independent nervous system. The information that originates in the heart is transmitted by this independent system through the vagus nerve to the thalamus to be processed by the amygdala and the hippocampus, which in turn transmit this data to the cerebral cortex. The amygdala, the reservoir of emotional memory, compares this new data to old before assigning it an emotional meaning and then determining the appropriate action with the help of the cortex.

Transformed into nervous impulses, heartbeats stimulate the electrical activity of the cerebral centers involved in the cognitive and emotional process. They form a language that influences the brain in assimilating information, making decisions, and storing experiences and expressing them creatively. Thus, the heart acts upon our perceptions and our reaction to the world.

Experiments have also shown that synchronization of emotion and thought improves mental clarity and imparts a feeling of well-being. Positive feelings optimize the functioning of the autonomic nervous system, the immune system, and the hormonal system and promote general brain efficiency. Altering the emotional state by concentrating on relaxing the heart transforms its effects on the forebrain and on the way the experience will be stored in memory.

Neurological Communication between the Heart and the Brain

The facing plate illustrates the interconnections among the vagus nerve, heart, and brain.

The information transmitted by the heart is essential to the proper functioning of the physical, emotional, and mental brain. This is why the heart is not merely a sensory organ but can actually be considered to have its own brain: the heart brain.

The heart communicates with the brain through the fibers of the central nervous system. These fibers enter

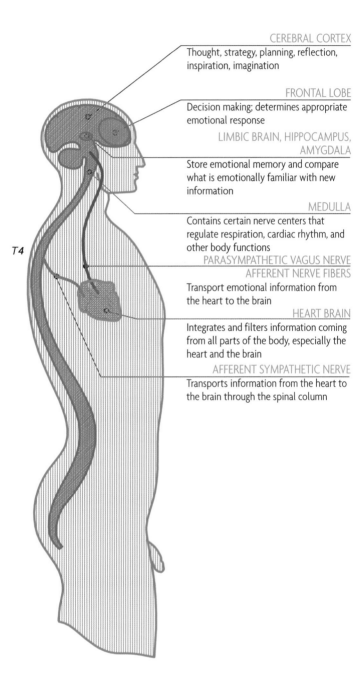

CEREBRAL CORTEX
Thought, strategy, planning, reflection, inspiration, imagination

FRONTAL LOBE
Decision making; determines appropriate emotional response

LIMBIC BRAIN, HIPPOCAMPUS, AMYGDALA
Store emotional memory and compare what is emotionally familiar with new information

MEDULLA
Contains certain nerve centers that regulate respiration, cardiac rhythm, and other body functions

**PARASYMPATHETIC VAGUS NERVE
AFFERENT NERVE FIBERS**
Transport emotional information from the heart to the brain

HEART BRAIN
Integrates and filters information coming from all parts of the body, especially the heart and the brain

AFFERENT SYMPATHETIC NERVE
Transports information from the heart to the brain through the spinal column

T4

the skull by way of the medulla oblongata, then ascend through the limbic brain and the hippocampus, which integrate emotions, decisions, and reasoning.

The nervous system of the heart (or heart brain) includes sensory fibers. They surround it and react to emotions, influencing its rhythm, as well as blood pressure and the secretion of hormones and neurotransmitters.

Intelligence Quotient (IQ) and Emotional Quotient (EQ)

At the beginning of the twentieth century, the results of IQ tests revealed that there was no significant increase in this figure from childhood into adulthood, no matter what quality of education was received. Intelligence was then considered to be innate and unalterable.

In 1985, Howard Gardner published the results of his studies on the numerous forms of intelligence. The human being possesses several types of intelligence: logical and mathematical, spatial, musical, kinesthetic, interpersonal (knowledge of others), and intrapersonal (self-knowledge). During this same period, John Mayer described the emotional intelligence that permits the individual to experience his relationships with others and to be aware of his thoughts and feelings as well as those of others.

Thus, the emotional quotient (EQ) was instituted. This tool offered a measure of the ability to recognize and express emotions. These are qualities necessary for understanding others and the way they function and for maintaining satisfying relationships with no tendency toward dependence or dominance. A satisfactory EQ demonstrates that the subject can work out her emotional problems and better manage her stress.

In his book *Emotional Intelligence,* Daniel Goleman brought out the fact that, unlike the IQ, the EQ can increase over the course of a lifetime. This explains why there are people of high IQ who seem to be failures, whose emotions are beyond them, sweeping them along and overwhelming them completely, whereas others with more average IQs have succeeded quite nicely.

If you wish to lead a balanced life, learn how to make full use of your emotional intelligence and learn to introduce civility into group situations, where misunderstandings among people so often rule their relationships.

The Functioning of the Heart's Intelligence

Negative emotions, such as sorrow and anger, destabilize the nervous system. They have a harmful effect on the cardiac rhythm and, in the long term, on overall health. Positive emotions, such as cheerfulness and love, bring harmony to the heartbeat, stabilize the nervous system, reduce stress, and encourage an optimistic view of the world around us.

By concentrating mentally on the heart with pleasant thoughts, one can balance its rhythm and thus play a positive role, through the agency of the autonomic nervous system, on the neurological and biochemical reactions that govern all the organs of the body. The activity of the sympathetic nervous system decreases, while that of the parasympathetic system increases.

Experiments were conducted in which the employees of a large corporation were encouraged to make use of their heart's intelligence. This brought about a reduction in—if not an outright elimination of—problems like insomnia, depression, autoimmune diseases, and anxiety.

Remember: The fetus possesses a beating heart and an emotional brain long before it develops a thinking brain.

The Memory of the Body

The human body is endowed with an infallible memory. The body does not forget and cannot lie.

The human tissue on which this memory is recorded is the fascia. Present throughout the body, from head to toe, the fascia envelops the muscles, the bones, the organs, the spinal cord, the arteries and veins, the rachidian nerves, and the cerebrospinal fluid. The fascia separates the various muscles by forming partitions between them, but it also keeps them connected in a pattern much like a spider's web. It consistently transmits tensions or movements from the moment it is stimulated.

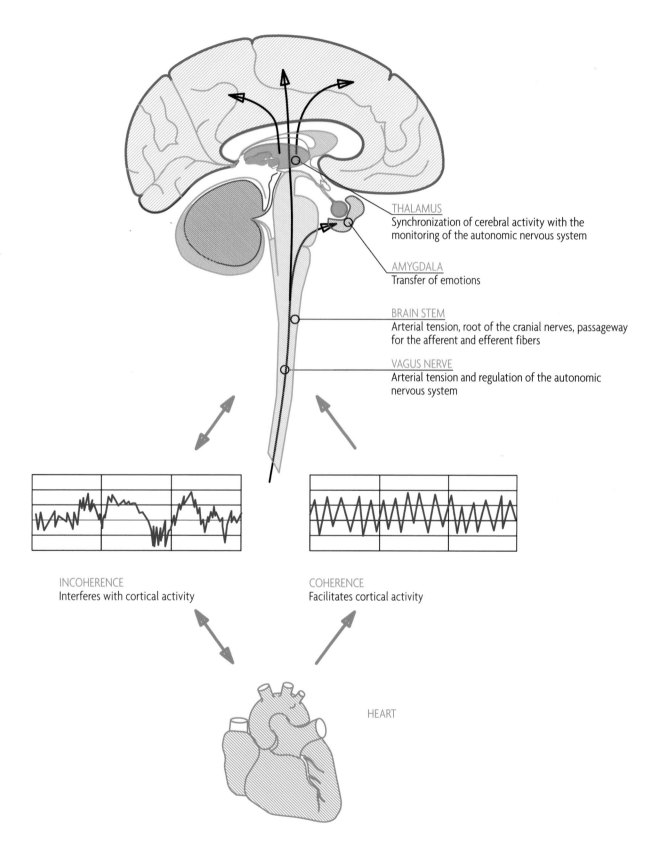

THALAMUS
Synchronization of cerebral activity with the monitoring of the autonomic nervous system

AMYGDALA
Transfer of emotions

BRAIN STEM
Arterial tension, root of the cranial nerves, passageway for the afferent and efferent fibers

VAGUS NERVE
Arterial tension and regulation of the autonomic nervous system

INCOHERENCE
Interferes with cortical activity

COHERENCE
Facilitates cortical activity

HEART

All the fascia is connected; the slightest tension on any level whatsoever will reverberate throughout the body. By means of this tissular chain, the fascia supports the body's defenses and plays a role in the regeneration of tissues and the elimination of toxins. But it creates dysfunctions from a distance in different organs by means of the autonomic nervous system and the endocrine system.

As indicated by its name, all connective tissue creates connections. This is true for any kind of connective tissue, including supportive tissue and even hematopoietic tissue—lymph nodes, the spleen, and bone marrow. From the outermost surfaces of the body to its deepest regions, all these layers build one upon one another and overlap.

The various fluids—plasma, lymph, serous fluids, and craniosacral fluid—circulate through the different compartments of the body thanks to the fascia. Circulation can occur from the extracellular environment to the intracellular because of the dynamic contractibility of the fascia and an elasticity that allows for constant movement.

When someone experiences an emotional shock, the body's tissues feel the tension, which then becomes imprinted upon the fascia. According to John Upledger, the tissue forms aqueous cysts or energetic cysts, which remain present even during dissection.

The emotional memory is the keeper of all the suffering an individual has ever experienced. This suffering forms the basis for how he or she approaches life; it goes into the unconscious and must be brought back out by a variety of methods so that emotional freedom can be reestablished.

Through the massage of the reflex points on the feet, reflexology can, by clearing away tensions, bring an emotional memory back to consciousness. The deepest layers of fascia hold records of memories going back to infancy; the more superficial layers hold memories of more recent experiences.

Here is when the therapist will see Hering's law prove itself true. During the different phases in a course of reflexology treatments, patients will remember dreams, forgotten sensations, sorrows, grief, and poorly assimilated experiences that have been recorded but never expressed and which they need to relive both physically and in their subconscious.

Foot reflexology treatments bring a sense of emotional freedom for many patients. They therefore often relive memories long forgotten through old symptoms that reappear, whose original function was to annihilate emotional memory; it is often unclear why working a certain zone should trigger these memories.

Foot reflexology, like osteopathy and all other natural therapies, follows this rule: the elimination from the inside toward the outside. The symptoms of the present gradually vanish and tend to bring about the resurgence of past symptoms. Moving backward through symptoms (from present to past) allows the emotional memories to be released from the body's tissues and be truly healed.

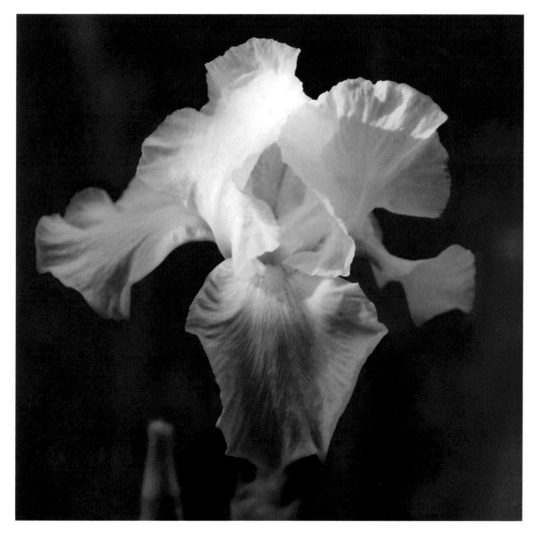

Iris

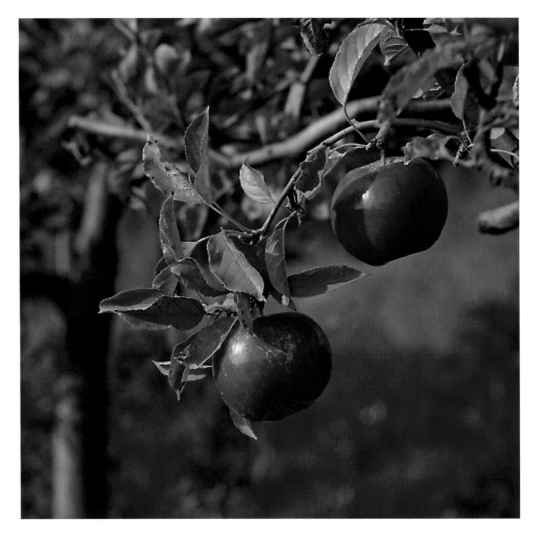

Life's simple pleasures

Life's Simple Pleasures Are the Best Therapy

In 1946 the World Health Organization (WHO) defined health as "a condition of complete physical, mental, and social welfare." Now, more than a half century later, while we are not sick as often or as long as people were sixty years ago, whatever happened to this welfare?

Let me simply remind the reader that physical activity develops the body, that life's pleasures cause the senses to bloom, that art and culture cause the mind to flourish, and that these things together, through their harmonious interplay, conspire to bring good health. This is one way to define the "healthy lifestyle."

Conversely, when we suffer life as if it were a burden, our health deteriorates on the three inseparable planes of the physical, the emotional, and the mental; in consequence, our social life falls apart as well.

The greatest healer is taking pleasure in living. Therefore, in order to bear the adversities and misfortunes that are, regrettably, inevitable, it is absolutely imperative that we nurture ourselves with pleasures, both great and small.

All too often, good health is presented as the culmination of a long and tedious effort consisting of many sacrifices, thankless physical exercises, and constant vigilance. But a wholesome lifestyle is first and foremost about revealing to the senses the pleasures that are often forgotten or unappreciated. The reeducation of the senses—or, even more accurately, their education—occurs through what are commonly called "life's simple pleasures."

The worst prison is the one that an individual constructs around himself. The way out is through the senses, the perpetual source of pleasures, and the dialogue they create with the outside world. Sight, hearing, smell, taste, and touch, ever satisfied anew, bring about a state of health and well-being.

No remedy, no technique, no healthy lifestyle can replace the joy of living. Life is the great healer. Welcome it as a priceless gift. Welcome the bliss of being, the great good fortune of tasting all of life's pleasures for the sheer joy of being alive.

Diet and Health

In the sixteenth century, Ambroise Paré defined dietetics as "the second half of medicine, which relieves illness through a good manner of living."

The Impact of Food on Health

It was Molière who declared that "one should eat to live and not live to eat." Our diet and way of life have changed radically over the past fifty years. The variety and quality of foodstuffs available initially contributed to lengthening the average life span, but today modern production methods, sedentary lifestyles, and dietary habits too rich in calories, sugar, salt, and harmful fats have created serious health risks: the rates of obesity, diabetes, cardiovascular diseases, and cancer are constantly increasing.

The origin for numerous pathologies can be found in a poor-quality diet. Large-scale international epidemiological studies, for example, have shown that a number of cancers are related directly to the dietary habits of different countries. Furthermore, the intense use of pesticides and fertilizers—outside of the fact that they poison the water, the fruits, the vegetables, and the livestock or human beings who eat them—depletes the soils so that the minerals and vitamins essential for health are disappearing from our foods.

The way one eats is just as important as what one eats. Meals should take place in a good atmosphere that feels lighthearted and calm. Chewing food peacefully helps the body to assimilate it well. If mealtime is stressful, this can cause hyperacidity. Stress compromises the oxygenation, combustion, assimilation, and elimination processes. The first stage of assimilation occurs through saliva, which is secreted at the mere mention of a dish that speaks to the senses. Saliva is indispensable to all digestive processes; therefore, food must be chewed for a long time.

Nutrition

Health is determined by the proper combination of nutrients in the diet.

Carbohydrates

The concentration of carbohydrates in the bloodstream equals one gram per liter; each day the brain consumes around 130 grams. The muscles draw their energy from glucose. The fetus draws the major part of its energetic needs from glucose as well.

The liver and the kidneys are almost exclusively in charge of glucose intake and distribution. Carbohydrates should make up 50 percent of a diet; insufficient amounts will create an imbalance in vitamins, minerals, and fibers. Complex carbohydrates—pasta, whole-grain breads, and legumes—should be prioritized; they soothe hunger and provide the energy needed for an entire day. Simple carbohydrates (such as refined sugar) cause the secretion of insulin, which increases the storage of fat.

Proteins

A basic building block of the cell, protein is present in varying quantity in almost all foods. Legumes are much richer in proteins than are grains. Eggs, dairy products, meat, and fish have the optimum biological value for protein consumption. The daily minimum intake should be around seventy grams.

Lipids

Lipids have the role of storing energy. A structural unit of cellular membranes, they serve as precursors for hormones, as cellular mediators, and as vehicles for liposoluble vitamins. They are supplied by meats (triglycerides rich in saturated fatty acids), fish (unsaturated fatty acids), and vegetables (mono- and polyunsaturated fatty acids).

Saturated molecules are rigid in contrast to unsaturated molecules, which are flexible and can easily insert themselves into cellular membranes. There, they play an essential role in the transmission of messages between neurons.

Linoleic and alphalinoleic acids, which are essential for cerebral functioning, are not synthesized by the body. They contribute to the building of biomembranes, whose numerous functions they ensure, and also take part in the production of messenger hormones. Linoleic acid is found in nuts and grapeseed, sunflower, corn, soy, and canola oils, and is indispensable on the neurobiological level, as all brain cells require a significant quantity in their composition. Linoleic acid also oversees the enzymatic activity of the brain. Saturated fatty acids (those found in meats) play a significant role in obesity, cardiovascular diseases, and colon and breast cancer.

Antioxidants

In the prevention of high cholesterol, vegetable fats are preferable to animal fats. The antioxidant micronutrients (vitamins A, C, and E) reduce the accruing of plaques responsible for arteriosclerosis. Vitamin C (along with flavonoids) makes the blood vessels less permeable, thereby preventing the infiltration of cholesterol. Polyphenols, selenium, and copper also possess antioxidant qualities. They work in synergy with the enzymes and the antioxidant systems of the cells to neutralize the activity of free radicals.

Fiber

Fiber comes from plants and has a beneficial effect on the digestive system, as it improves intestinal transit. Working with numerous minerals, it slows the absorption of lipids and carbohydrates, thereby keeping energy from building up too quickly. Fiber facilitates the elimination of cholesterol and encourages nitrogen excretion in the stools by absorbing biliary salts, thereby providing relief to the kidneys as well. It seems to improve the healing of colon cancer and to facilitate the absorption of magnesium and calcium. Fruits, vegetables, grains, and legumes all contain significant quantities of fiber.

Vitamins

A varied diet is important for providing the body with the vitamins it needs to function properly. Nevertheless, self-medication with supplements should be avoided, as it can cause liver congestion and hyperacidity in the stomach, which lead to fatigue and weight gain. The body can store only two vitamins as reserves: vitamins A and D.

Mineral Salts and Trace Elements

Mineral salts and trace elements are essential for chemical and enzymatic exchanges and reactions. A deficiency will cause significant health problems. They are present in the body in infinitesimal amounts and consequently should not be administered without supervision, as imbalances may result.

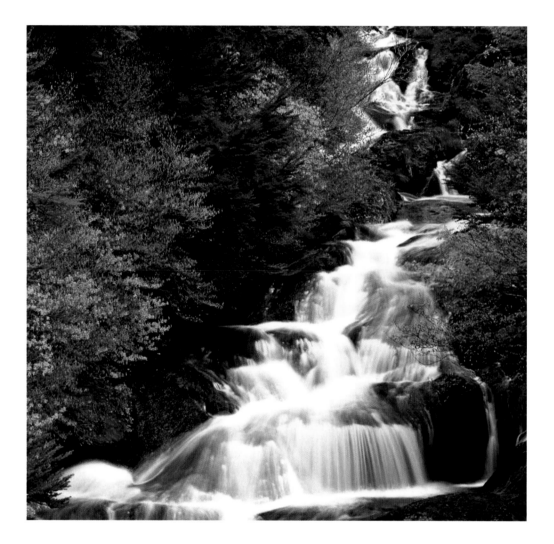

The Healing Power of Water

Millions of people are suffering from diseases caused by the insufficient absorption of water. Pathologies such as asthma, diabetes, arthritis, angina pectoris, obesity, Alzheimer's disease, high cholesterol, and high blood pressure are signs of distress from the body pointing to water deprivation. The book *Your Body's Many Cries for Water,* by Dr. Fereydoon Batmanghelidj, shows that the majority of degenerative diseases can be avoided if we drink enough water on a daily basis.

Held as a political prisoner in a Tehran prison starting in 1979, Dr. Batmanghelidj was surrounded by men who were suffering for the most part from stomach pains brought about by stress and who were lacking any medical assistance or medications. He observed that a glass of water was enough to bring relief to prisoners bent double by acute gastric pains.

Once released from prison, he began conducting research on the use of water as medicine. This work would lead, some twenty years later, to the publication of his bestselling book. Specialists have since confirmed the effectiveness of the methods he put forth, which no doubt could make for incalculable savings in the health budgets of nations as well as families.

The Role of Water in Metabolism

Water is the most indispensable substance for the proper functioning of our bodies. Dehydration is the starting point for numerous physiological disorders. In fact, daily intake of water is essential not only for the proper physical functioning of the body but for maintaining optimum emotional and mental states as well.

People may believe that thirst is an alert signal that precedes dehydration. This is not the case. When thirst manifests, dehydration is already under way; the disorders it has engendered then require some two to three liters of water per day for several weeks to restore the tissues to their proper balance with no other medication. Fatigue, depression, sadness, and discouragement then give way to a feeling of well-being.

Humanity at its earliest origins comes from an aquatic species. The human being's body is composed of 75 percent water or aqueous fluid. Since the day of creation, the role played by water has not changed. Human beings owe a good part of their life to water. This is at once a legacy and a dependency.

In crisis situations (fear, for example, brings thirst) or in dehydration, the body prioritizes the vital organs, giving its water reserves to their irrigation. This rationing process will endure for as long as the body experiences water as scarce; it ceases as soon as the body's water balance has been restored. All bodily functions adapt to this rerouting of water so that vital nutrients can reach the high-priority organs and enable them to overcome states of stress. This mechanism contributes to survival as part of the fight-or-flight process governed by the sympathetic nervous system.

Today this "reflex" rationing is increasingly triggered in the body because of the hectic pace of life in the modern world. It is crucial for people to drink water often.

The control of water distribution in the body is in service to the vital importance of the organs whose survival it ensures. Of these, the brain comes first. It represents 2 percent of total body weight but is irrigated by 18 to 20 percent of the body's blood circulation, whose flow will fluctuate depending on the brain's activity.

It is a mistake to believe that drinks like tea, coffee, alcohol, and sodas can replace water. To the contrary, in order to absorb these synthetic liquids, the body needs an even greater quantity of water; thus, drinking them has the consequence of further reducing the body's natural water reserves. A state of dehydration will then become established in the body's bone, muscle, joint, mucosal, and glandular structures.

Today's children drink lots of fruit juice and sodas loaded with sugar, preservatives, and food dyes instead of drinking water. It is deplorable that doctors are not doing enough to alert their patients to the primordial clinical role played by water.

Despite the signs of distress given off by the body (thirst, dryness), the correlation between dehydration and the deterioration of certain bodily functions is rarely established. The harmful effects of dehydration can be far-reaching, to the point of affecting someone's descendants. Its symptoms are, unfortunately, most often silent. When these symptoms do manifest, people often try to silence them with painkillers that aggravate the physiological effects of dehydration in the cells and tissues even more. Children and the elderly are the most at risk. Doctors and patients both should take into account the role played by dehydration in migraines and in cardiac, rheumatic, and vertebral ailments, as well as in digestive pains, especially from colitis and constipation.

In order to make progress in this domain, it is essential that people understand the basics of dehydration. Life is born of water. The body consists of 25 percent solid matter and 75 percent fluids. These fluids include transport agents, such as blood and lymph; lubricants, such as mucosal secretions and the synovial secretions of the joints; conductors, such as extracellular fluid; and secretors, such as digestive juices.

Water intake should equal the amount of liquid expelled as urine. The kidneys, along with the liver and the pancreas, are the first to be stricken by the injurious effects of dehydration and can degenerate to a point that is irreversible.

Gastric Pains and Constipation

Heartburn, gastritis, and duodenitis are the first signs of chronic dehydration. When ulceration occurs, a water cure must be followed; if this does not bring about immediate relief, then surgery is the next recourse. In the case of ulcers, perforation, and abdominal rigidity accompanied by acute pains despite medication, water consumption must be increased. A glass of water reaches the intestines in three minutes.

The digestion of solid foods requires a great deal of water. The mucus of the stomach and intestines is 98 percent water. When water intake is insufficient, it will be drawn from the body's reserves at the digestive system's expense. A glass of water drunk half an hour before mealtime will help the stomach absorb solid and acidic foods.

Pain at the bottom left side of the abdomen (the lower part of the intestine) is often a sign of dehydration. The primary cause for constipation is dehydration. Even appendicitis has been known to dissipate with three glasses of water!

Motilin, whose secretion depends on the absorption of water, has the role of stimulating peristalsis, the contracting of the intestines, and the opening of the sphincters from one end of the digestive tract to the other; this explains its direct effect on constipation. It also serves to signal the feeling of satiety.

The pyloric sphincter is a valve that opens to allow the stomach's contents to pass through. Reverse peristalsis occurs when this valve contracts instead of relaxing. Acidic stomach fluid then flows back toward the esophagus, causing heartburn. This is gastroesophageal reflux, which can result in a hiatal hernia. Lying down right after a meal exacerbates this problem.

Water is essential for all the digestive functions. For example, the pancreas secretes a bicarbonate solution that prepares the upper portion of the intestines to receive the stomach acids and reduces their corrosive effects. Furthermore, the more water one drinks, the greater the amount of fluid that collects in the intestines and the more the blood volume goes up.

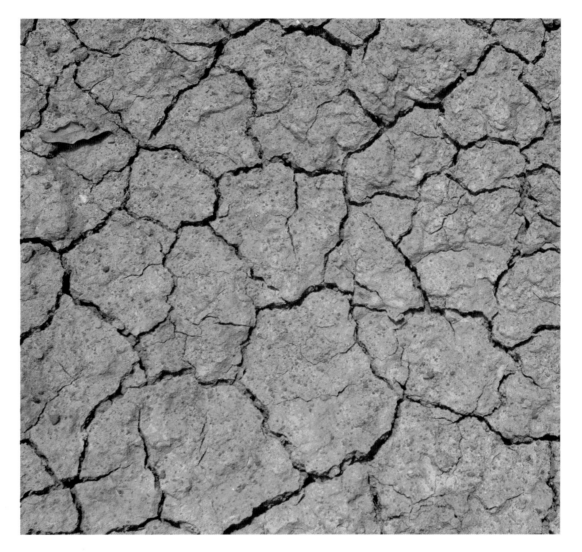

Aridity

Pathological Conditions Due to Lack of Water

Rheumatism and Arthritis

Bone cartilage contains a considerable amount of water, and its lubrication is dependent upon this fluid. Well-hydrated cartilage is protected from friction and abrasion. Inside the bone marrow, the manufacture of blood cells is dependent upon water. The dilation of the blood vessels, which is encouraged by water, improves circulation within the bone tissue.

Joint pains that are due to the destruction of the joint surfaces can often be relieved by sufficient intake of water. This will enable the production of the hormones responsible for rebuilding these tissues.

Lumbar and Cervical Pains

Disks and vertebrae require lubrication, especially when the disks have suffered compression. Seventy-five percent of the body's weight is supported by the volume of water contained in the center of the vertebral disks; the other 26 percent is supported by the fibrous material surrounding these disks.

A slowly occurring cellular dehydration will keep the vertebral cartilage from regenerating. This can lead to juvenile arthrosis; it also contributes to the phenomenon of aging. Any treatment aiming to correct injuries caused by poor posture should be accompanied by the ingestion of two to three liters of water per day.

Mobility, which is essential to good blood circulation, is often hampered by pain. The painkillers often prescribed to address this problem will, as we noted earlier, cause dehydration; this should be compensated for with plenty of water. It is equally advisable to increase water consumption before and after any physical exercise.

Angina Pectoris

Drinking copious amounts of water along with the proper diet will lower blood cholesterol levels in three weeks. Cholesterol stops up the arteries and constricts them, the result of which is insufficient irrigation of the muscles. This will require three liters of water per day, to ensure a gradual and thorough rehydration.

Headaches

Dehydration is one of the major causes of headaches, due often to variations in temperature caused by dysfunction of the liver and kidneys. Rehydration, which is essential in any case for overall circulatory needs, is a priority for anyone taking medication, which only aggravates the body's existing lack of water. The same is true during periods of stress.

Stress and Depression

A prolonged state of stress will cause the brain to consume too much water. It has been observed that negative thoughts and feelings, such as sorrow and fear, reduce the body's water reserves. A state of crisis results because the hormones secreted during stress (endorphins, cortisol, prolactin, vasopressin) only accentuate the need for water, often without the individual's awareness. Endorphins prepare the body to endure a period of fatigue or a state of fear until the stress that caused them has disappeared.

Cortisol mobilizes stored energy, converting fats into acids and proteins into amino acids. Burned as fuel by the muscles, these fats also serve to form neurotransmitters. If the action of the cortisone is prolonged, the body's reserves of water and amino acids will be depleted. Sugars are burned away first under the cortisol's influence, after which the body must nonetheless continue to feed on its reserves in response to the urgent need at hand, such as fighting an infection. In prolonged states of stress, this phenomenon can thus cause irreparable damage to the tissues.

Tumors

Chronic dehydration can lead to the development of breast tumors. Persistent and increasing secretion of prolactin can change the glandular tissue of the breasts into precancerous tissue—and even cancerous. The risk is increased by hereditary factors and by stress, in particular. Regularly drinking plenty of water reduces any

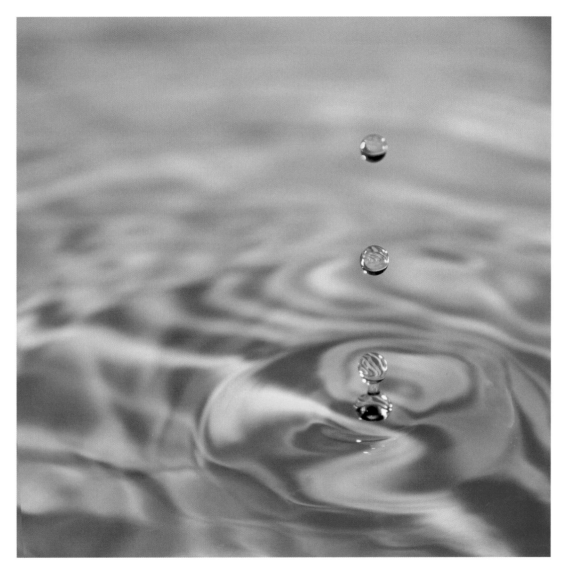

Water

predispositions to breast cancer; this is equally true for men and prostate cancer.

Water and Pregnancy

During pregnancy, 75 percent of the volume of the dividing cells is made up of water. This ensures the growth of the placenta and the production of amniotic fluid. Water is also indispensable for the production and development of the fetus. Milk production in the mammary glands is stimulated by prolactin (which also stimulates the reproductive organs), and water is the principal component of breast milk. In the event of stress or dehydration, the body's priority will be to ensure the survival of the child, at the mother's expense.

Alcohol, Tea, and Coffee

Many people on a daily basis drink coffee, tea, or even alcohol instead of water. This increases dehydration in the body and deprives the nervous system of the water it needs—with a staggering reduction in nerve activity.

Caffeine, moreover, is an inhibitor of the equilibrium of phosphates, which are essential to eyesight and memory. Caffeine must therefore be strictly prohibited for children who show any signs of trouble with their schoolwork. Older people with Alzheimer's disease should drink nothing but water.

Alcohol reduces the secretion of vasopressin in the pituitary gland; this brings about a state of general dehydration, but especially in the cells of the brain, which will then be unequipped to handle stress. The ingestion of alcohol also causes excessive amounts of endorphins to be produced by the body. Because endorphins can be addictive, regular consumption of alcohol can easily lead to addiction. As women have a tendency to secrete more endorphins (during lactation, menstruation, and pregnancy), three years is enough for them to become addicted. For men, it takes seven years for addiction to set in.

Obesity

While walking and exercising are indispensable, to fight against obesity it is even more crucial to drink extra water. The brain translates the body's needs for energy or water into cravings: hunger and thirst. But it is quite common for people to mistake thirst for hunger, which leads them to eat when their bodies are crying out for water. Dehydration is even implicated in compulsive eating: just after eating, thirst is often mistaken for continued hunger. By making it a habit to drink a glass of water before every meal, you can learn to distinguish the two sensations and avoid overeating.

Artificial Colorings and Sweeteners

Artificial colorings and artificial sweeteners (aspartame, saccharine, sucralose, and others) hyperstimulate the cells of the brain, liver, kidneys, pancreas, and endocrine glands. Absorbed by the body much more quickly than natural products, they prompt exaggerated cerebral activity, as well as excess activity in the cells of the other organs. Conversely, natural sugars that are more slowly metabolized yield a normal physiological effect. Body chemistry cannot withstand lengthy periods of processing unnatural products without a toll on its essential functions. Excessive stimulation of the brain also heightens the sensations of thirst and hunger.

In order to metabolize sugar, the liver manufactures glucose from other nutritional substances taken in by the body. The absorption of artificial sugars consequently overtaxes the liver, which must work harder to break them down into forms that the bloodstream can absorb. Even more serious, artificially sweetened foods and drinks are addictive. Ninety minutes after their ingestion, because of the insulin discharged in the bloodstream in response to the food or drink, a resurgence of hunger occurs, demanding immediate attention. They also stimulate the cellular reserves and thereby prompt further weight gain.

Water and Cerebral Activity

The brain consumes a significant quantity of energy. It requires strong and plentiful blood circulation, which in turn requires the right amount of water intake. The process of digestion produces about 20 percent of the

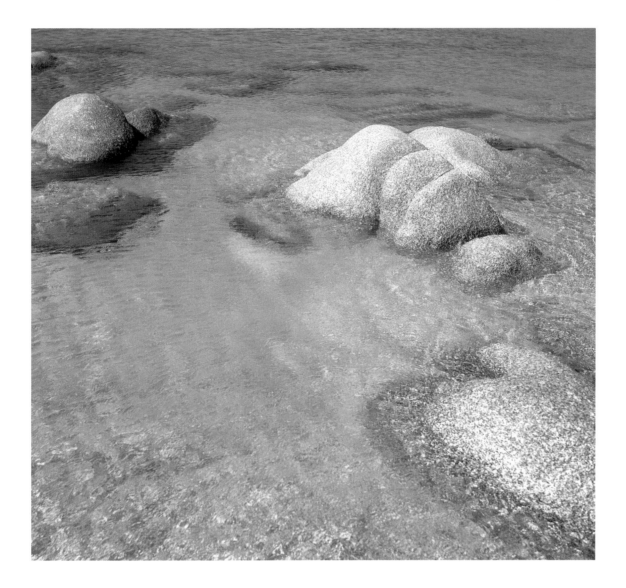

brain's energy needs, and it draws additional energy from fat, muscle, and tissue. However, the hydroelectric energy conversion of water remains the primary source of energy for the brain.

Any form of stress will cause dehydration.

Asthma and Allergies

Histamine is a neurotransmitter that regulates the bronchial muscles. It is also antibacterial and antiviral and eliminates any agents that are foreign to the body. It also performs a chemical action on proteins. When the body's water levels are normal, its action remains imperceptible; but its effects increase when either mild or severe dehydration sets in.

In the case of asthma or allergies, its level increases in these muscles, causing them to contract in an exaggerated manner. The loss of water through natural evaporation is then reduced because of these bronchial contractions. However, this in no way calls for reducing water intake, as water is crucial to heal this pulmonary condition. Plenty of water will allow the histamine levels to go down in three to four weeks and the allergic reaction to disappear. A certain amount of salt is also important for asthmatics because it is a natural antihistamine with antimucosal effects.

Vasopressin

Vasopressin is a polypeptidic hormone that regulates the gradual and selective intake of liquids—and thus, of water—to certain cells of the body. The pituitary gland secretes the vasopressin that travels through the general circulatory system. Specific receptors exist in the cells to receive this vasopressin, which serves to prevent cellular dehydration. Each receptor transforms into a filter, or sodium pump, and the water absorbed by the cell then travels through the cellular membrane to change into blood. In maintaining the activity of the receptors, vasopressin ensures a regular flow of fluids through all the body's systems, especially the nervous system.

In the event of severe dehydration, vasopressin will control and even ration the distribution of water. But it is ineffective in chronic dehydration cases, whose symptoms often reveal an emergency situation that hasn't been detected in time.

Renin-Angiotensin

Headquartered in the kidneys, the renin-angiotensin system (RAS) plays a central role in the control of the body's fluid volume. It is subordinate to the action of histamine, which, as we have seen, also regulates water absorption.

Set into motion by histamine activity in the brain and kidneys, the RAS goes into action when the body's total volume of fluids diminishes. Intended for the retention of water, it stimulates the absorption of both water and salt and returns to its normal rate of activity only when they return to normal levels.

The RAS also causes the capillaries of the vascular system to constrict. The constriction of the blood vessels is actually measurable and is better known as blood pressure. In stressful states, blood pressure rises, and water is used for the transformation of proteins into glycogenic substances and fats. When there is a lack of renin-angiotensin, the vessels tighten up.

Vascular constriction or high blood pressure was not sufficiently recognized in the past as the signal for loss of fluid or dehydration. The excess activity of the RAS will come to a halt only with the ingestion of enough water and salt to bring about normal vascular constriction.

To sum up, dehydration is the primary pathogenetic agent in the human body and in all living cells. The high blood pressure and excess cholesterol that are responsible for the majority of heart attacks are themselves caused by dehydration. Pure, clear water that satisfies all the body's fluid needs cannot be replaced in any way by chemical substitutes.

Traveling back through the history of the biological evolution of living creatures, we now know that humans, like all other mammals, are beings born of water. It is therefore quite logical that this "natural habitat" would play a fundamental role in the human body and brain; we must absolutely take in, each and every day, a sufficient amount of this chemical mediator of life.

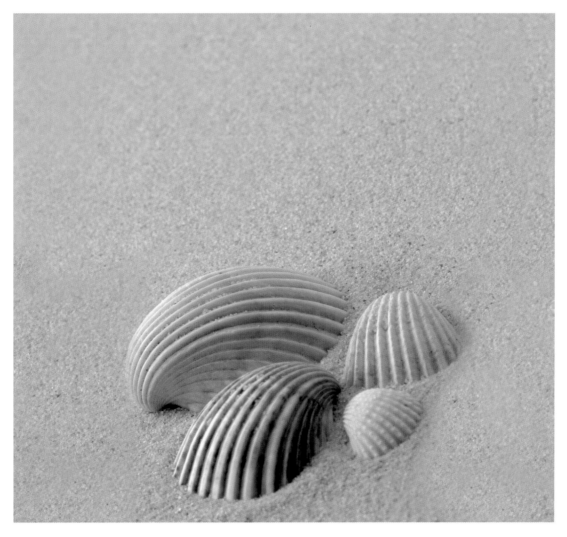

Venus before her birth

The Exquisite Hour

The white moon
Shines through the trees:
From every branch
There springs a voice
Beneath the leaves . . .

O my beloved.

Like a deep mirror
The pond reflects
The silhouette
Of the black willow
Where the wind is weeping

It is the time, let us dream

A vast and tender
Assuagement
Seems to be falling
From the firmament
Made iridescent by a star.

It is the exquisite hour

PAUL VERLAINE, *La Bonne chanson*

PART FIVE

Total Reflexology Therapy

The Occipital Zones and the Ten Reflex Zones

The occipital zones are located on the back of the head on the lower part of the occiput, arranged laterally between the mastoidal sutures and the occipital protuberance. The ten side-by-side vertical zones of the feet and hands are tightened up to be laid out between the occiput and the upper level of the ear. Each zone can be treated on the three horizontal occipital zones: the structural, the sympathetic, and the parasympathetic. These are important to give attention to in all pathological conditions brought on by stress. The occipital zones are exact reflections of all the body's organs and structures.

The occipital reflex zones permit the reflexologist to decode the autonomic nervous signals from the thalamus that are given off by the reticular nucleus (of diagnostic importance), balance the body through reflex massage (of therapeutic importance), and establish a direct correlation with the reflex zones on the hands and feet.

The Horizontal Occipital Reflex Zones

The horizontal occipital reflex zones are made up of three bands corresponding to different areas. The lower band corresponds to the physical structure of the body. The middle band corresponds to the sympathetic nervous system. The upper band corresponds to the parasympathetic nervous system.

The lower boundary of the rectangle formed by these three bands is the horizontal plane supported by the atlas (vertebra C1), while the lateral boundaries are the occipitomastoidal sutures. The area of this rectangle is where the reflexologist can locate the precise point that corresponds to the part of the body affected by the illness or disorder at hand. Here, too, is where one can determine whether it is internal, structural, emotional, or mental in nature.

The Vertical Occipital Zones

The three vertical occipital zones coincide with three of the main reflexology zones. The innermost zone coincides with reflexology Zone One and provides information about the movement, blockages, and rate of the cerebrospinal fluid. The middle zone overlaps with Zone Three and gives information about the energetic activity, blockages, or harmonious functioning of the hormones. The outermost zone coincides with Zone Five and indicates blockages in lymphatic activity.

The pressure applied to the reflex points here, using the pad of the thumb, should be light; this allows the practitioner to feel energy blockages (crystals, tensions, depression). In order to avoid making the patient dizzy, it is important to stop at the mastoidal suture and not go lower than the foramen magnum or the atlas.

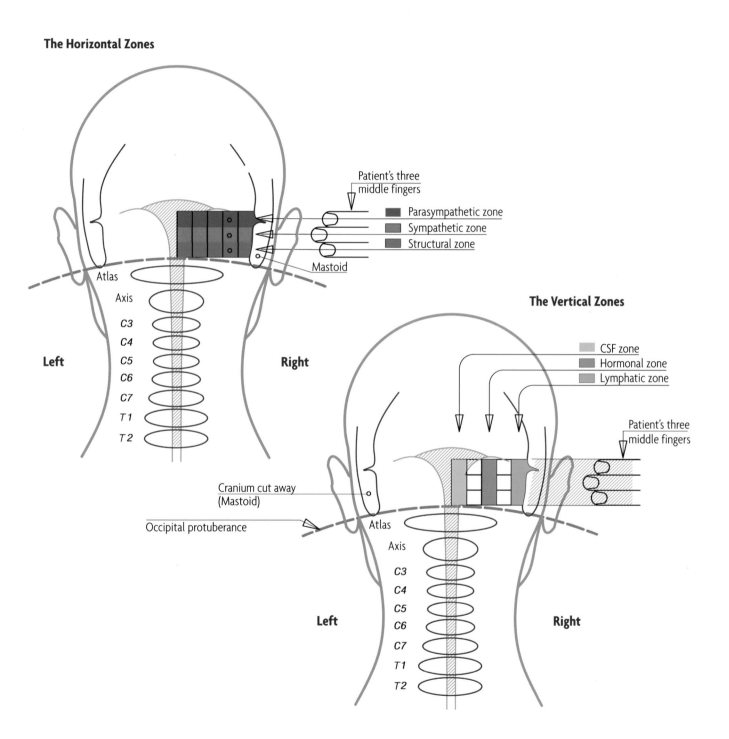

The Horizontal Zones

Patient's three middle fingers

Parasympathetic zone
Sympathetic zone
Structural zone

Mastoid

Atlas
Axis
C3
C4
C5
C6
C7
T1
T2

Left

Right

The Vertical Zones

CSF zone
Hormonal zone
Lymphatic zone

Patient's three middle fingers

Cranium cut away (Mastoid)

Occipital protuberance

Atlas
Axis
C3
C4
C5
C6
C7
T1
T2

Left

Right

The Craniosacral System

Bringing the craniosacral system into reflexology is of fundamental importance because a great number of patients suffer from disorders and illnesses connected to some cranial trauma that has in turn created structural damage to the body. In the majority of cases, this trauma goes back to birth. Dr. Viola Frymann, who examined 1,250 newborns, found that only 11.6 percent did not show any cranial distortion.

Typical childhood diseases, migraines, sterility, and, notably, the deterioration brought about by aging all respond well to cranial therapy. Numerous psychiatric ailments originate from trauma affecting the occipitomastoidal sutures, the sphenobasilar synchrondrosis (SBS), and the frontosphenoidal and ethmoidal sutures. This trauma can also lead to physical degeneration.

Brain Physiology

The skull is perforated with numerous orifices: on the front, where the nerves that connect to the sense organs—sight, hearing, smell, and taste—pass through; at the base of the cranium, where the cranial nerves, arteries, and veins pass through; and finally, on the level of the occipital foramen, where the spinal cord passes through.

The volume of the brain and the spinal cord is approximately 1,650 milliliters, of which 150 milliliters is taken up by the CSF. The CSF is both a liquid and a nerve and is thus able to transmit the brain impulses that govern all functions in the body. This fluid is contained in the ventricles of the brain, in the cerebral cisterns or ventricles that are located beneath and around the brain, in the subarachnoid space (which descends from the brain to follow the spinal column), and in the spinal cord, all the way down to the sacrum. This network of containers holds the fluid that protects the central nervous system. (For more, see the plate Circulation of the Cerebrospinal Fluid, page 75.)

The CSF is regulated to maintain a level of constant pressure. Thus, it serves the brain as a kind of shock absorber inside the cranium. By diffusing, feeding, and cleansing the nervous system cells, it nourishes all the structures of the brain and the spinal cord. It acts as a filter and an aspirator. It transports hormones and peptides. As the fluidic protector of the brain, it works in harmony with the other fluids of the body, such as blood and lymph. It is a chemical and physical protective agent and consequently contributes to the transmission of emotional and mental nervous impulses between cells. Through its pH, it influences the primary respiratory mechanism (PRM), or cerebral respiration, and, indirectly, pulmonary respiration. If the pH is too acidic, physiological cellular exchanges will not take place.

The osteopath William Sutherland discovered the PRM in 1933 and perfected the technique that permitted its modification. He observed that in the central nervous system and all its dependent structures there is a rhythmic movement (flexing and extending) that can be broken down as follows:

- ▶ Movement of the sutures connecting the twenty-nine bones of the cranium
- ▶ Expansion and contraction of the cerebral hemispheres (a flexing and extending movement)
- ▶ Movement of the membranes enveloping the spinal cord and the brain
- ▶ An undulating movement in the CSF that bathes the spinal cord and the brain
- ▶ An involuntary movement of the sacrum directly connected with the flexing and extending move-

The Cranial Diaphragm
Seen in Three-Fourths Profile from the Back

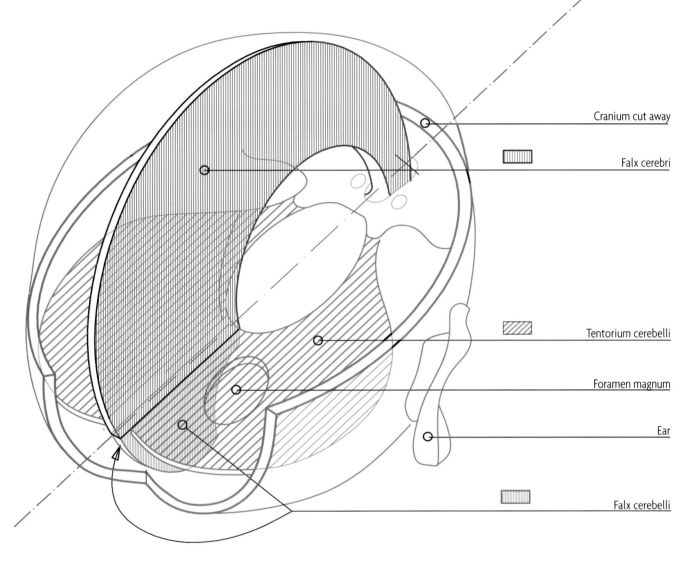

Cranium cut away

Falx cerebri

Tentorium cerebelli

Foramen magnum

Ear

Falx cerebelli

ments of the cranium via the spinal column and the spinal cord and its membranes

The body's homeostasis is dependent upon this PRM, with the central nervous system regulating both voluntary and involuntary effects (the autonomic nervous system) throughout the body. When information is received, brain function is triggered by the perception of electromagnetic and sound waves translated into electrical impulses. The CSF and its flexing and extending movement are the result of a rhythmic pumping activity directed by the glial cells of the brain. The CSF receives electromagnetic information, which it retains in memory. It transmits this information throughout the body by means of the spinal cord.

In sensorial activity, neuronal oscillations create a network of interactions. These complex waves are picked up by the cells, broken down into simple waves, and translated into electrical impulses (cellular memory).

The brain vibrates at various frequencies, both harmonious and non-harmonious. The pineal gland serves as the central point for the emission and reception of these vibrations. Bones, membranes, and fluids play the role of sound box and selective amplifiers. The quality of this "music" depends on numerous factors: the quality of the sense organs (transmitters); the state of the neurons and the brain (the richness of the intra- and interhemispheric connections); cellular marking and reverberation (acquired or transmitted memory, previous choices, and "learning" experiences); resonance quality of the skull, whose shape, plasticity, and density alter the interference fringes; holographic reconstructions from simple waves; quality of the frequencies picked up (scales, coherence, intensity); and the subject's motivation and attention—primary functions of consciousness.

Information is shared, in the vibratory mode, by all parts of the brain and, therefore, simultaneously, by all parts of the body.

Damage to the Primary Respiratory Mechanism (PRM)

Damage to the primary respiratory mechanism can manifest in many ways throughout the body, by either changes in the rhythm, volume, fluctuation, composition, and circulation of the CSF; changes in the structure, position, or freedom of movement of the bones; or changes in the structure or function of the meninges, nerve passageways, or fascias.

The causes of damage to the PRM are many and varied. Trauma can create compensatory alterations in the spinal column or skull or a reflex effect of an irritation in some distant part of the body. Environmental factors can create serious psychological trauma. Prenatal or natal events can lead to primary, insidious bone lesions, including secondary lesions on the level of the soft tissue or a primary lesion in a joint membrane from a sudden, traumatic birth.

The Reflexology of the Brain

Reflexology provides access to every structure inside the skull. By working on the membranes of the brain, the dura mater, the arachnoid, the pia mater, the falx cerebri, and the tentorium cerebelli, the practitioner can improve memory and offer relief for Alzheimer's disease, phobias, and so forth. (See pages 125 and 128–29.)

The big toes provide a reflection of the entire brain, with the right hemisphere on the right foot and the left hemisphere on the left. This includes the neocortex, the limbic and reptilian brains, the hippocampus, the amygdala nuclei, and the mammillary tubercles. The two cerebral hemispheres communicate information to each other through the corpus callosum. (See page 136.)

Human Memory

Several zones of the brain are involved in the process of memorization. The temporal lobe of the cerebral cortex is where long-term memory is located. The putamen is where the "memory procedure" necessary for learning new things—for example, how to ride a bicycle—is stored. The hippocampus has the function of holding on to reference points and relocating the winding paths that lead to memories of past events. The amygdala is the headquarters for unconscious, emotional, and traumatic memory. The caudate nucleus is the headquarters for instinct and the genetic code.

Reflex pressure activates the circulation of blood, lymph, and the cerebrospinal fluid. Reflexology can stimulate or calm. Its balancing and normalizing effect has a positive influence on the physical body, the psyche, and different states of consciousness.

The Cranial Nerves

1. The Olfactory Nerve (sensory)
Territory concerned: nasal fossae
Function: smell
Disorder: anosmia (loss of the sense of smell)

1a. The Gustatory Nerve (sensory)
Territory concerned: mucous membranes
Function: taste
Disorder: ageusia (absence of the sense of taste)

2. The Optic Nerve (sensory)
Territory concerned: eyes; muscles of ocular globe, of eyelid, of retina
Function: sight
Disorder: anoopsia (misalignment in which both eyes are deviated upward)

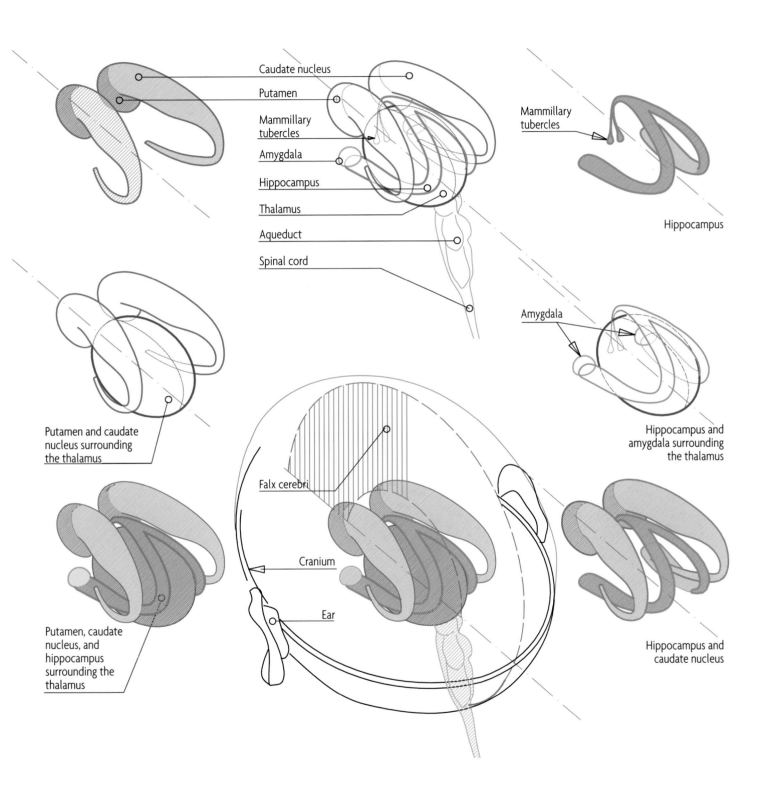

Caudate nucleus

Putamen

Mammillary tubercles

Amygdala

Hippocampus

Thalamus

Aqueduct

Spinal cord

Mammillary tubercles

Hippocampus

Putamen and caudate nucleus surrounding the thalamus

Amygdala

Hippocampus and amygdala surrounding the thalamus

Falx cerebri

Cranium

Ear

Putamen, caudate nucleus, and hippocampus surrounding the thalamus

Hippocampus and caudate nucleus

3. Oculomotor Nerve (mixed function, primarily motor)

Territory concerned: eyes, muscles of ocular globe, lifter of the upper eyelid; four extrinsic muscles

Functions: movement of the eyelid and the ocular globe, accommodation of the crystalline lens for near sight, constriction of the pupil, muscular sensitivity

Disorders: ptosis (drooping eyelid), strabismus (misalignment of the eyes), loss of accommodation for near sight and diplopia (double vision)

4. Patheticus (or Trochlear) Nerve (mixed function, primarily motor)

Territory concerned: superior oblique muscle

Functions: movement of ocular globe and muscular sensitivity

Disorders: diplopia, strabismus

5. Trigeminal Nerve (mixed function)

Territory concerned: eyes; maxilla and mandible; face, forehead, teeth, sinuses, salivary glands, nose, mouth, tongue, soft palate

Functions: mastication, painful and thermal sensations in the territories concerned, muscular sensitivity

Disorders: paralysis of the muscles used for mastication, loss of thermal and tactile sensations, tics, trigeminal neuralgia

6. Abducens Nerve (mixed function, primarily motor)

Territory concerned: right lateral muscle

Functions: movement of the ocular globe and ocular sensitivity

Disorder: convergent strabismus

7. Facial Nerve (mixed function)

Territory concerned: outer ear (concha); muscles of the face, scalp, and neck; tear glands; sublingual, submandibular, nasal, and palatine glands

Functions: tears and saliva, facial expression, muscular sensitivity, taste

Disorders: facial paralysis, ageusia

8. Vestibulocochlear Nerve (sensory)

Territory concerned: inner ear, vestibular branch

Functions: hearing, balance

Disorders: tinnitus, deafness, vertigo, ataxia, nystagmus (involuntary eye movements)

9. Glossopharyngeal Nerve (mixed function)

Territory concerned: parotid glands; carotid sinus and stylopharyngeal muscle; the rear third of the tongue, larynx, and tonsils

Functions: salivary secretion, taste, and regulation of blood pressure; muscular sensitivity

Disorders: difficulty swallowing; reduction in saliva production, loss of sensitivity in the throat; ageusia

10. Vagus Nerve (mixed function)

Territory concerned: tongue, tonsils, larynx, pharynx, inner and outer ear, heart, lungs, bronchial tubes, stomach, small intestine, part of the colon, gallbladder, and glands of the digestive tract

Functions: contraction and relaxation of the smooth muscles, release of digestive substances, sensations originating in the organs concerned, and muscular sensitivity

Disorders: swallowing difficulties, paralysis of the vocal cords, loss of sensitivity in the organs involved

11. Spinal Accessory Nerve (mixed function, primarily motor)

Territory concerned: larynx, pharynx, soft palate, foramen lacerum; cervical, sternocleidomastoid, and trapezius muscles

Functions: swallowing, muscular sensitivity, head movements

Disorders: paralysis of the sternocleidomastoid muscle and the trapezius, absolute inability to turn the head or lift the shoulders

12. Hypoglossal Nerve (mixed function, primarily motor)

Territory concerned: all the muscles of the tongue

Functions: tongue movement, muscular sensitivity

Disorder: trouble with mastication, speech, and swallowing

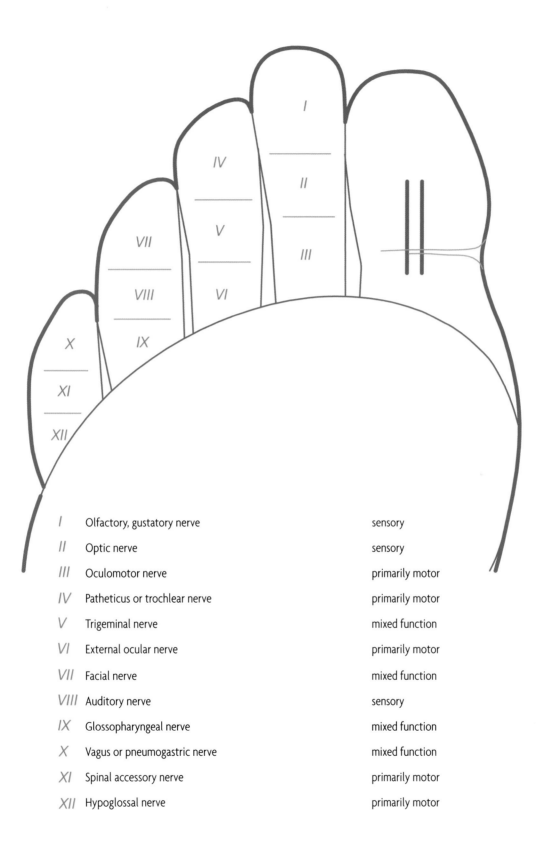

I	Olfactory, gustatory nerve	sensory
II	Optic nerve	sensory
III	Oculomotor nerve	primarily motor
IV	Patheticus or trochlear nerve	primarily motor
V	Trigeminal nerve	mixed function
VI	External ocular nerve	primarily motor
VII	Facial nerve	mixed function
VIII	Auditory nerve	sensory
IX	Glossopharyngeal nerve	mixed function
X	Vagus or pneumogastric nerve	mixed function
XI	Spinal accessory nerve	primarily motor
XII	Hypoglossal nerve	primarily motor

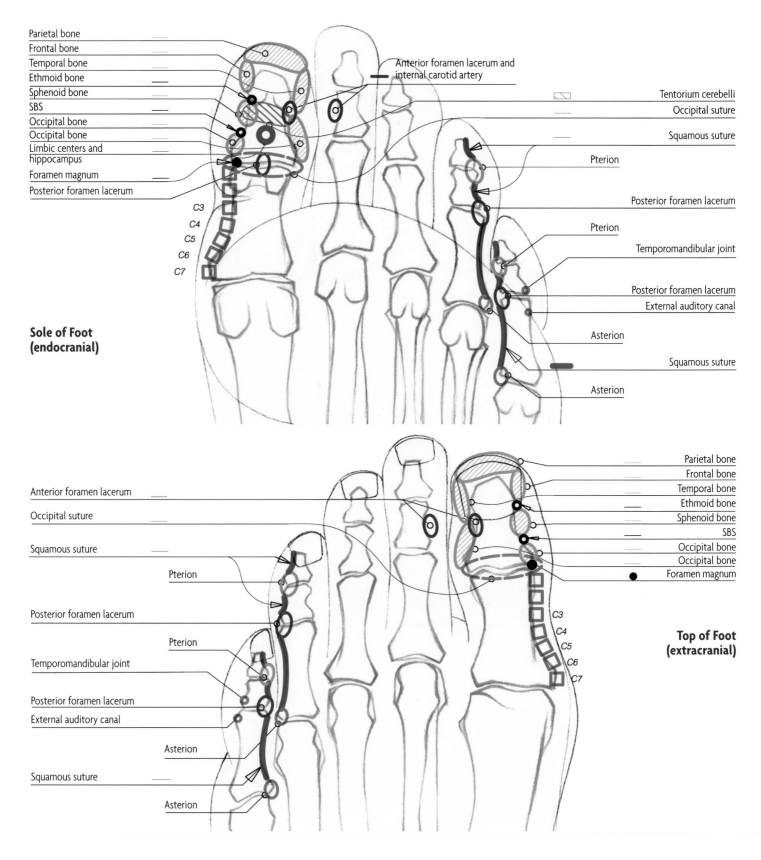

Parietal bone
Frontal bone
Temporal bone
Ethmoid bone
Sphenoid bone
SBS
Occipital bone
Occipital bone
Limbic centers and hippocampus
Foramen magnum
Posterior foramen lacerum

Anterior foramen lacerum and internal carotid artery

Tentorium cerebelli
Occipital suture

Squamous suture

Pterion

Posterior foramen lacerum

Pterion

Temporomandibular joint

Posterior foramen lacerum
External auditory canal

Asterion

Squamous suture

Asterion

C3
C4
C5
C6
C7

Sole of Foot (endocranial)

Anterior foramen lacerum

Occipital suture

Squamous suture

Pterion

Posterior foramen lacerum

Pterion

Temporomandibular joint

Posterior foramen lacerum
External auditory canal

Asterion

Squamous suture

Asterion

Parietal bone
Frontal bone
Temporal bone
Ethmoid bone
Sphenoid bone
SBS
Occipital bone
Occipital bone
Foramen magnum

C3
C4
C5
C6
C7

Top of Foot (extracranial)

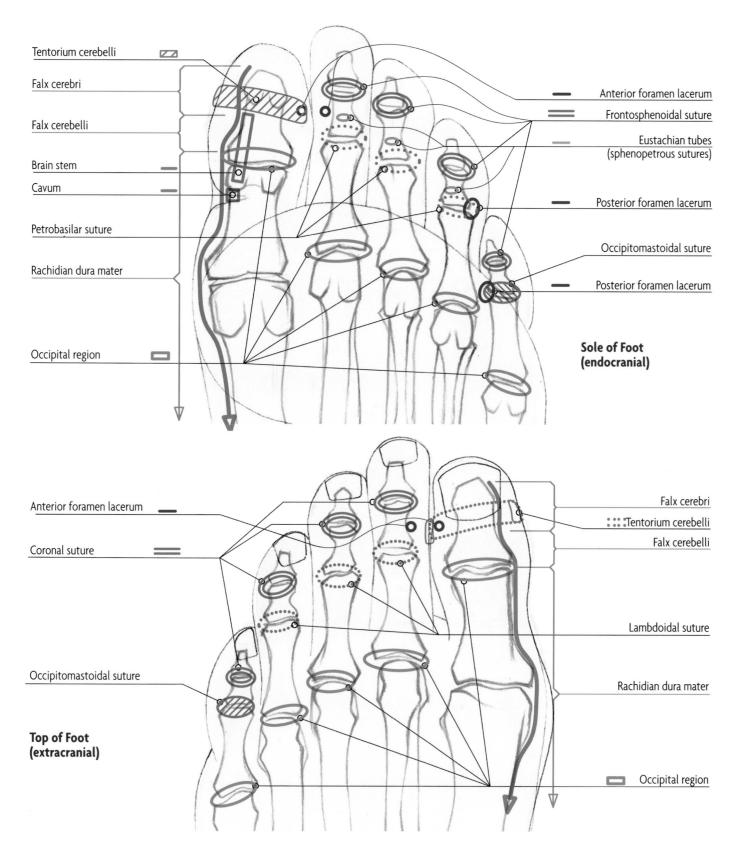

Tentorium cerebelli

Falx cerebri

Falx cerebelli

Brain stem

Cavum

Petrobasilar suture

Rachidian dura mater

Occipital region

Anterior foramen lacerum

Frontosphenoidal suture

Eustachian tubes
(sphenopetrous sutures)

Posterior foramen lacerum

Occipitomastoidal suture

Posterior foramen lacerum

**Sole of Foot
(endocranial)**

Anterior foramen lacerum

Coronal suture

Occipitomastoidal suture

**Top of Foot
(extracranial)**

Falx cerebri

Tentorium cerebelli

Falx cerebelli

Lambdoidal suture

Rachidian dura mater

Occipital region

Left Top of Foot

Right Top of Foot

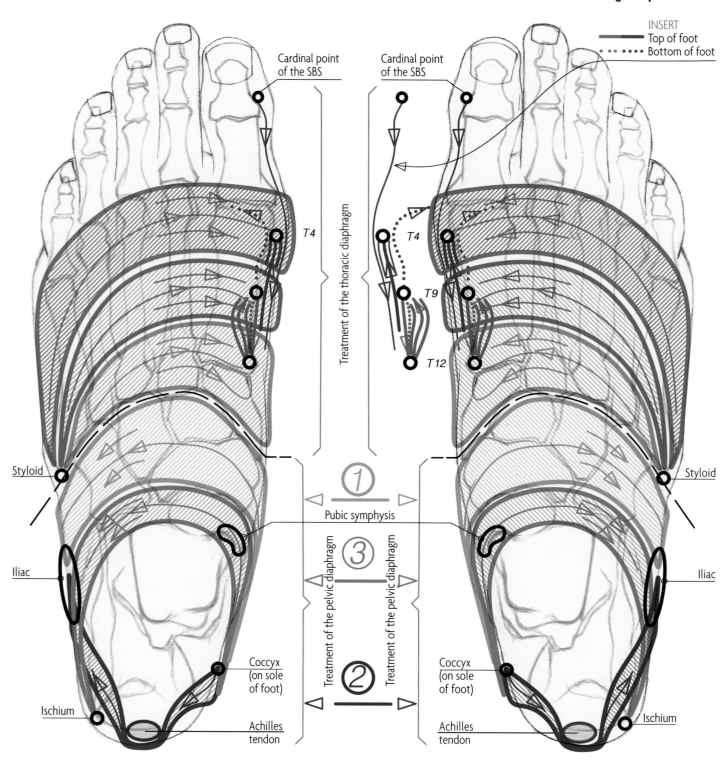

Cardinal point of the SBS

Cardinal point of the SBS

INSERT
Top of foot
Bottom of foot

T4

T4

T9

T12

Treatment of the thoracic diaphragm

Styloid

Styloid

① Pubic symphysis

③

Iliac

Iliac

Treatment of the pelvic diaphragm

Treatment of the pelvic diaphragm

②

Coccyx (on sole of foot)

Coccyx (on sole of foot)

Ischium

Ischium

Achilles tendon

Achilles tendon

The insert on T4, T9, T12 indicates the direction and the number of movements.

Reflexology for the Craniosacral System
The Organic Emotional Zones on the Center of the Foot

Right Sole of Foot

Left Sole of Foot

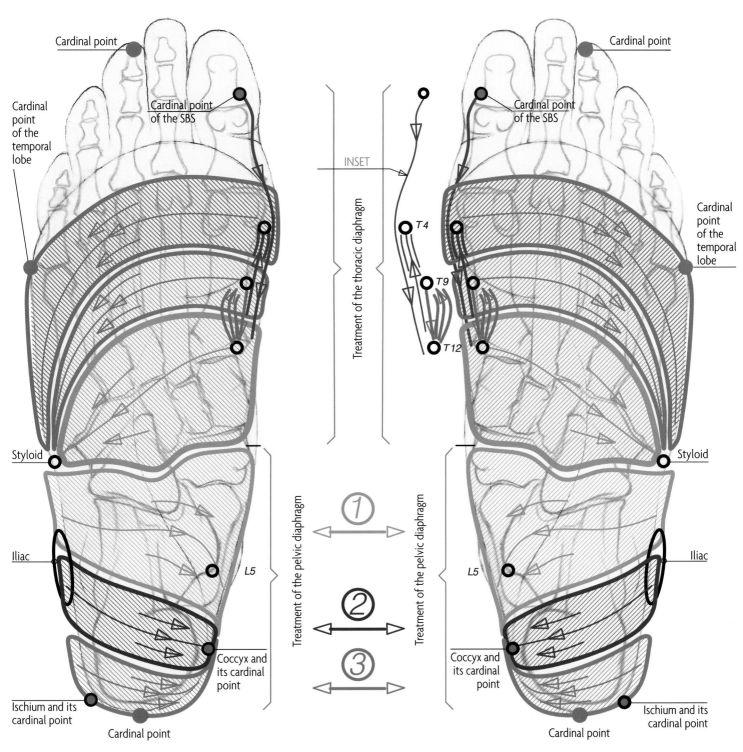

Cardinal point

Cardinal point of the SBS

Cardinal point of the temporal lobe

Styloid

Iliac

L5

Coccyx and its cardinal point

Ischium and its cardinal point

Cardinal point

INSET

Treatment of the thoracic diaphragm

T4

T9

T12

Treatment of the pelvic diaphragm

① ←→

② ←→

③ ←→

Treatment of the pelvic diaphragm

Cardinal point

Cardinal point of the SBS

Cardinal point of the temporal lobe

Styloid

Iliac

L5

Coccyx and its cardinal point

Ischium and its cardinal point

Cardinal point

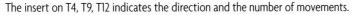

The insert on T4, T9, T12 indicates the direction and the number of movements.

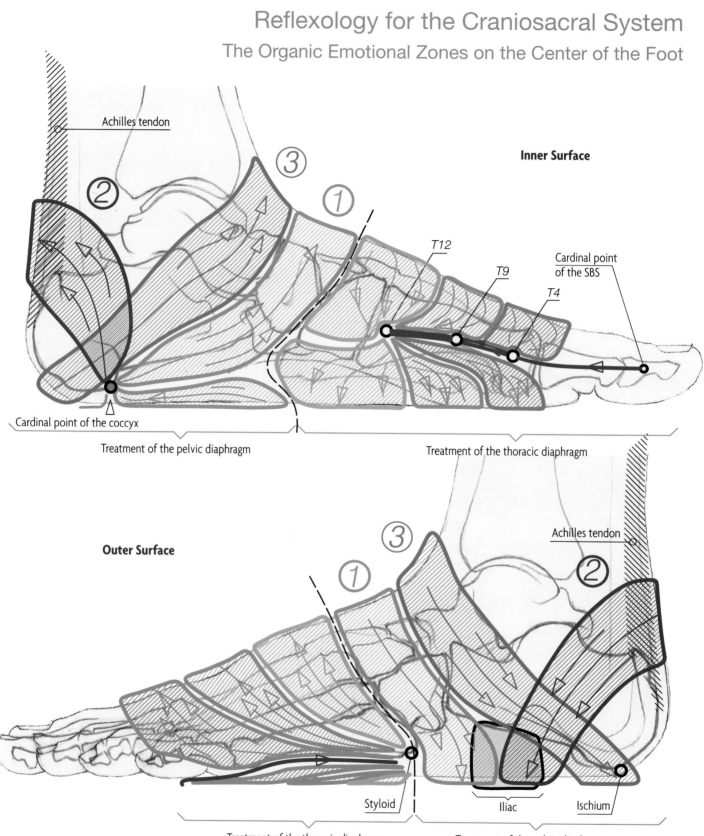

Inner Surface

Achilles tendon

T12

T9

Cardinal point of the SBS

T4

Cardinal point of the coccyx

Treatment of the pelvic diaphragm

Treatment of the thoracic diaphragm

Outer Surface

Achilles tendon

Styloid

Iliac

Ischium

Treatment of the thoracic diaphragm

Treatment of the pelvic diaphragm

The Organic Physical Zones
on the Center of the Foot
Pelvic Floor

Right Sole of Foot

Left Sole of Foot

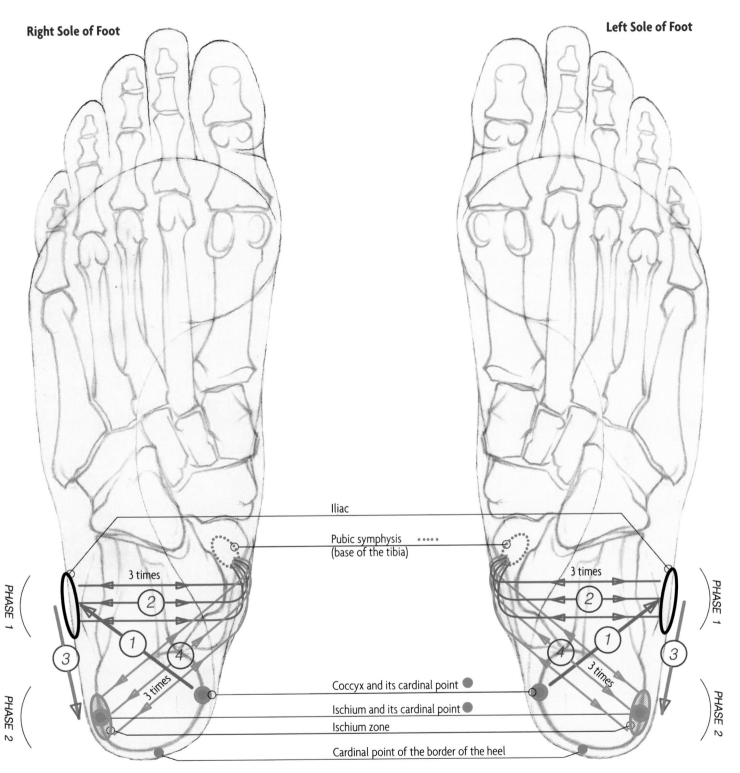

Iliac

Pubic symphysis
(base of the tibia)

3 times

3 times

PHASE 1

PHASE 1

PHASE 2

PHASE 2

3 times

3 times

Coccyx and its cardinal point

Ischium and its cardinal point

Ischium zone

Cardinal point of the border of the heel

The Craniosacral Approach
for the Heel of the Foot
Border of the Heel

Right Sole of Foot

Left Sole of Foot

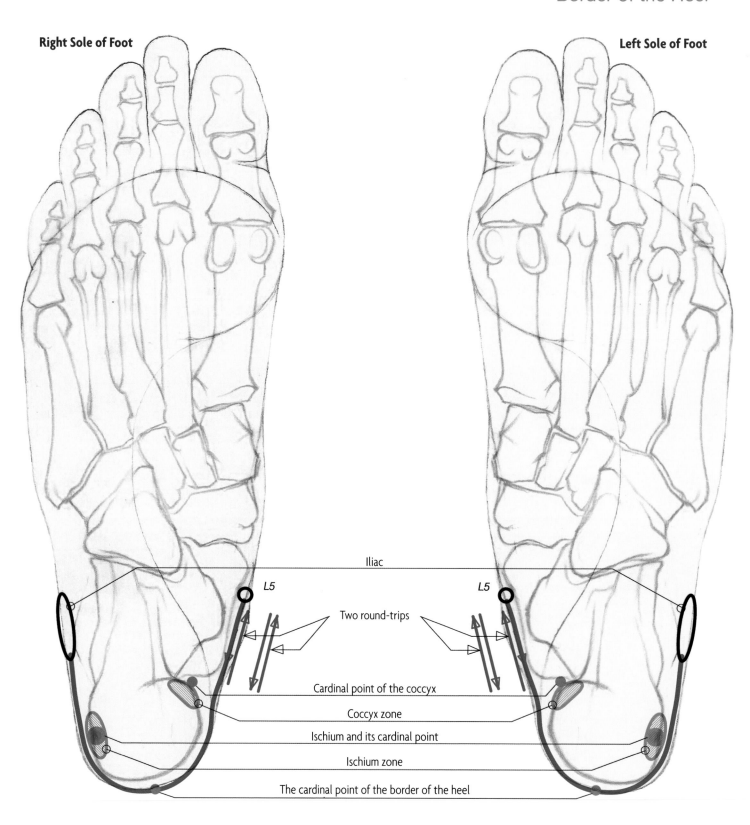

Iliac

L5

L5

Two round-trips

Cardinal point of the coccyx

Coccyx zone

Ischium and its cardinal point

Ischium zone

The cardinal point of the border of the heel

The Organic Physical Zones
on the Heel of the Foot
Pelvic Floor
Border of the Heel

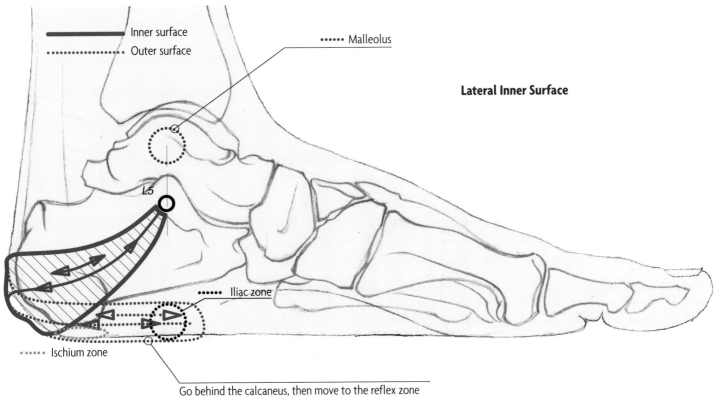

Inner surface
Outer surface

Malleolus

Lateral Inner Surface

L5

Iliac zone

Ischium zone

Go behind the calcaneus, then move to the reflex zone
of the ischium, then that of the iliac on the outer surface.

Sole of the Foot (endocranial)

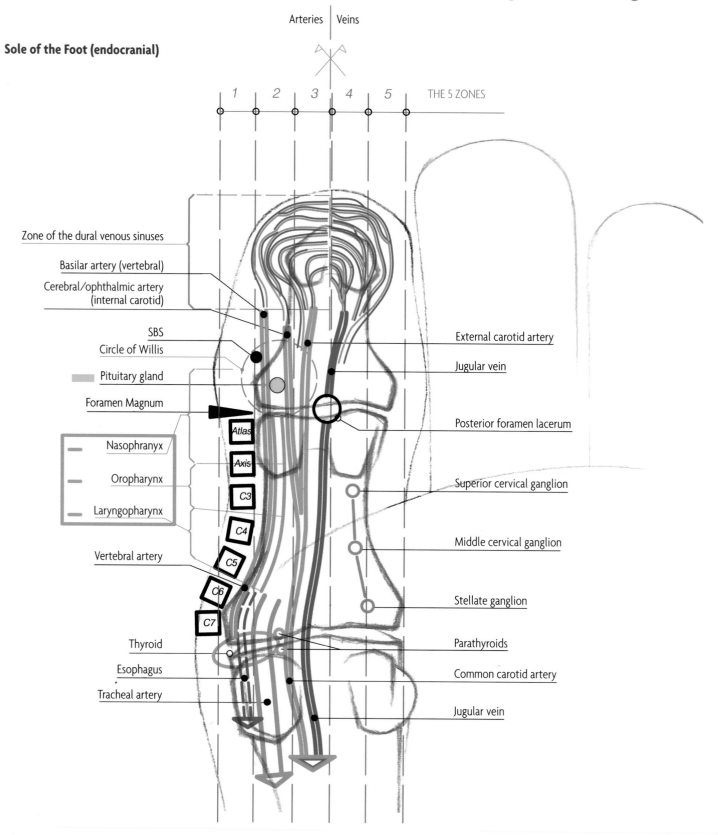

Arteries | Veins

1 2 3 4 5   THE 5 ZONES

Zone of the dural venous sinuses

Basilar artery (vertebral)

Cerebral/ophthalmic artery
(internal carotid)

SBS

Circle of Willis

Pituitary gland

Foramen Magnum

Nasophranyx

Oropharynx

Laryngopharynx

Vertebral artery

Thyroid

Esophagus

Tracheal artery

External carotid artery

Jugular vein

Posterior foramen lacerum

Superior cervical ganglion

Middle cervical ganglion

Stellate ganglion

Parathyroids

Common carotid artery

Jugular vein

Atlas

Axis

C3

C4

C5

C6

C7

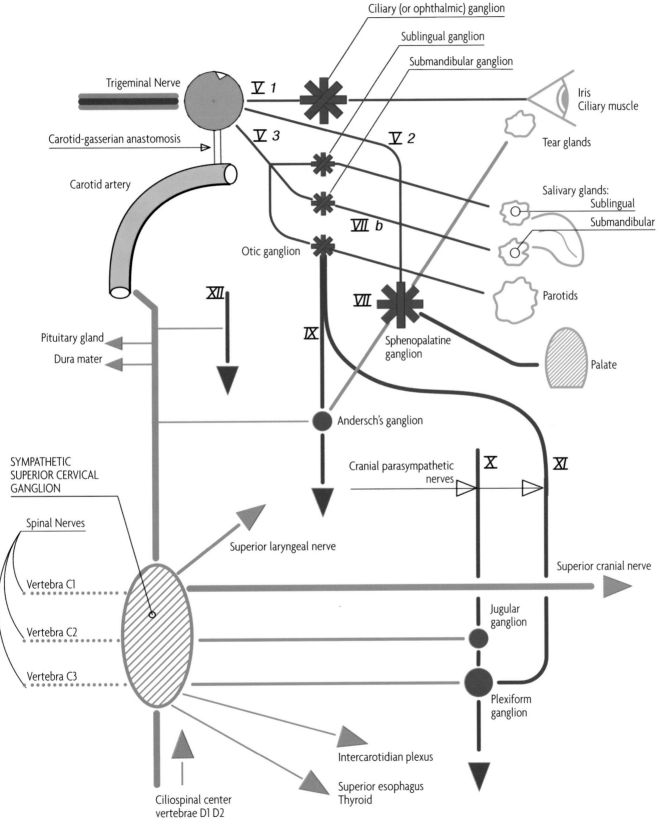

Stress Syndrome

The word *stress* originated in the English language and means pressure, tension, constraint, aggression. It is the body's response to a "stressor." Stress comes of two opposing forces (physical, spiritual, mental, social, temporal, etc.) that collide but cannot merge—no wonder tension results!

The first stress everyone undergoes is birth. A baby, whose nervous system will not be complete until the age of two, arrives in an environment of dazzling light and noise. She is touched by unknown hands and feels fear. These first impressions will leave a permanent imprint in her tissues, character, and entire being.

Stressors

Stressors vary from one person to the next, based on their past experience or on information they have been able to integrate at some time of life, either recently or in the most distant past. In any case, two individuals will not have the same interpretation of the same event, as each will experience—physically, emotionally, or mentally—in accordance with his own situation and in accordance with his values and personal memories.

Thought is a creative process. Since it is determined by the events we experience, both negative and positive, it is also receptive, enabling us to analyze these events. By this token, it determines the unfolding of our lives, just as it conditions our memories. Our response to stressors will therefore be an entirely individual one and will differ, based on our past and our nature, from that of, say, some hard-times companion going through the same event at the same time. There can be no typical response to any certain type of stressor.

This does not prevent us from analyzing a stressor's mechanical principles, so that we can understand how to restore balance with appropriate treatment. Still, the practitioner will need to base his or her diagnosis in each case on the personality of the patient—the general classification and multiple details that affect the person's physical, psychic, and mental makeup.

Stressors first of all bring about a biological response from the body. The body begins to secrete hormones that will allow it to adapt as it faces the new situation. This adaptation will essentially depend on the state the body is in at the onset of stress.

Stimuli

Physical stimuli: As mentioned above, the first stress everyone endures is a physical one: birth. Other physical stressors include fatigue, exertion, injury, and illness.

Chemical stimuli: These can include pollution, intoxication, drugs, anesthesia, and vaccines.

Sensory stimuli: Through sight: the spectacle of violence, overwhelming bright lights, ugliness, visual pollution. Through hearing: sporadic noises, such as explosions; continuous noise, such as a motor or an aggressive rhythm. Through touch: shock, sensations of hot and cold, sharpness, or aggressiveness. Through smell: strong odors. Through taste: strong flavors.

Social stimuli: Work, unemployment, being laid off, loneliness.

Climatic stimuli: Extremes in heat or cold, rain, snow.

Emotional stimuli: Fear, great joy (these stimuli can also be of a social or sensorial nature).

Psychoaffective stimuli: Parent-child conflicts, betrayals in love relationships, divorce, mourning; also, the absence of stimuli, loneliness, loss of one of the senses

Stressors can be negative when they bring about disease and a loss of vitality or positive when they stimulate one's motivation or creativity.

The Mechanisms of Stress

Thus, stressors stimulate the sensorial receptors—eyes, ears, nose, mouth, and skin—through the reflex arc. The stimuli travel through both the sympathetic and parasympathetic aspects of the autonomic nervous system. They climb from the hypothalamus to the thalamus, then to the limbic centers and the cortex. Hormonal relays take place at the level of the pituitary gland and the pineal gland. The neuroreceptors of the cells are informed by the CSF, blood, and lymph.

If the immune, nervous, and endocrine systems are affected by prolonged stress, the body will be thrown out of balance and homeostasis will be completely off-kilter. This will express itself through various physical symptoms and cellular disorders.

The Six Stages of Stress Syndrome

Stress causes disarray in both the sympathetic and the parasympathetic nervous system. With all the changes this brings about and the fatigue that ensues, the body ends up in a state of exhaustion. Stress, as noted earlier, involves the conflict between opposing "forces," such as two competing deadlines or the battle of your immune system against a virus.

The following stages then occur in sequence:

1. The body's difficulty in merging these two forces sets off the "alarm phase."
2. The "adaptation phase" is launched once merging has begun.
3. After the two forces have been merged in this adaptation, the disorder will have created a chronic loss of overall energy to ensure compensation to the vital organs.
4. If this state endures, either the sympathetic or the parasympathetic system will become weaker than the other, until chronic fatigue becomes acute.
5. This acute fatigue leads to the exhaustion of both systems.
6. Ultimately, life cannot be sustained and death results.

The Sympathetic System and Stress

Fear is a great example of what is at once an abstract feeling and also a physical rush of adrenaline molecules. Happiness is also expressed in the form of thoughts and elaborated on the molecular level.

Without hormones, then, feelings would not exist. The same is true for pain, which would not be felt without the signals of the neurons that transmit it. There would be no sensation of relief, either, without the endorphins that block the pain receptors. Everywhere a thought or feeling goes, there is a chemical substance accompanying it. Everywhere there is mental distress, some biochemical pathogenetic conversion occurs.

With the help of adrenaline, emotions travel at great speeds through the bloodstream. If they activate the receptors located in the cardiac cells, the rhythm of the heart will also be activated; the sympathetic nervous system will then be stimulated in turn. This chain reaction progresses in stages. The alarm phase is revealed by increased activity of the sympathetic nervous system.

What someone has experienced in life, the manner in which he or she overcame past ordeals, plays a crucial role in an extreme situation. The person who faced a trying event in the past and rose above it will, in the present, catch sight of the possibilities for survival. The event can be experienced positively through mental activity and reflection.

How to Fight Stress

According to Hering, all assimilation implies elimination, and elimination can be encouraged through reflexology; the stimulation of hearing (music), sight (soft light, harmonious shapes and colors, restful landscapes), taste (healthy foods and a balanced diet), and touch (massage); the oral expression of thought (psychotherapy); and expression through creative movement (dance, yoga, gymnastics).

The will to resist stress plays a major role. As the brain has the capability to regenerate, govern, and transform itself, it gives the body the right instructions for coming back to homeostasis. By replacing obsessive and negative images with images from positive past experiences, the reference points for all future experience are modified and future stress can be prevented or at least minimized.

Stress and Reflexology

Stress, acting through the receptors in the sense organs, imprints itself in the cortex and in cellular memory. It can then cause upheaval in the rhythms of sleep and disturb the general equilibrium of the body. Memories of an emotional nature are the most powerful on the cellular level.

Reflexology can help erase this cellular emotion by restoring harmonious circulation in the contracted tissues. The lymphatic glands are then able to perform their cleansing work. The movement of the lymph gently erases the imprint made by stress, and those minuscule points on the foot no longer testify to the poor nervous and hormonal functioning of the corresponding organ. The cleansing process of the lymph restores the body to balance, and stress is absorbed through the autonomic nervous system.

The behavior, words, and touch of the therapist can help the patient adapt to stress if the patient's energy permits it. When the practitioner finds "cords" or "crystals" on the foot, reflex massage becomes painful and often indicates a long-held stress or chronic disorder. It then helps to lighten the pressure and even move away from that area and come back to it later, again with a light touch.

Stress Syndrome on the Feet

		FUNCTIONAL STAGES		PHYSICAL STAGES	
		ALARM	ADAPTATION	CHRONIC STATE	EXHAUSTION
SIGNS AND SYMPTOMS		S.S.*	S.S. and P.S.†	P.S. ↗ for acute crisis	S.S. ↘ P.S. ↘
		Pain +++ No contraction Tissues are receptive to touch	Generalized pain that is not fixed to any one location +++ Contraction of tissues Hardening of tissues Granulation	Localized fixed pain +++ Contractions = cords Points sink deeper Hypersecretion	Pain that is not acute Limp feet
TREATMENT STRATEGIES		Working the P.S. • Cranial zones • Pituitary gland • Solar plexus • Adrenal glands • Sacrum • Calming	To be worked first: • The dorsal column (S.S.) • Solar plexus • End with the P.S.	For acute crisis, use general treatment For chronic states, treat S.S. +++	Light general treatment of S.S. and P.S.

*S.S. = sympathetic system

†P.S. = parasympathetic system

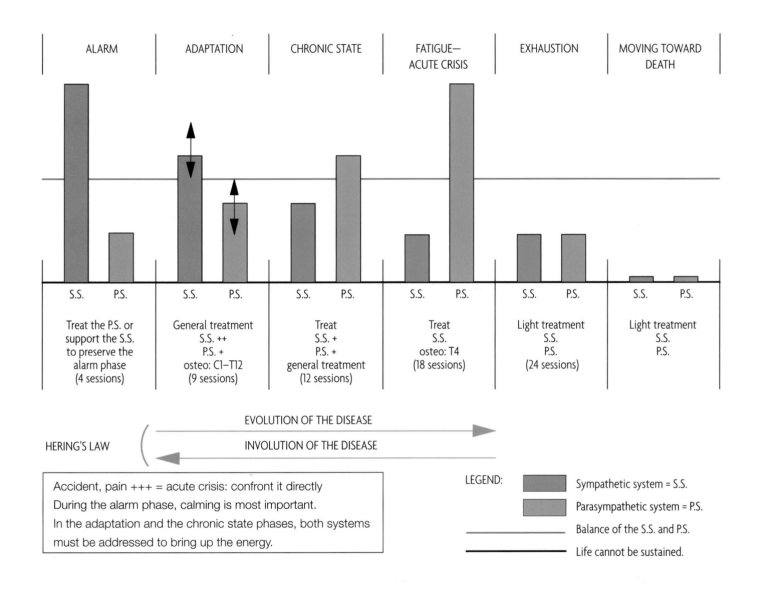

ALARM	ADAPTATION	CHRONIC STATE	FATIGUE—ACUTE CRISIS	EXHAUSTION	MOVING TOWARD DEATH
S.S. P.S.	S.S. P.S.	S.S. P.S.	S.S. P.S.	S.S. P.S.	S.S. P.S.
Treat the P.S. or support the S.S. to preserve the alarm phase (4 sessions)	General treatment S.S. ++ P.S. + osteo: C1–T12 (9 sessions)	Treat S.S. + P.S. + general treatment (12 sessions)	Treat S.S. osteo: T4 (18 sessions)	Light treatment S.S. P.S. (24 sessions)	Light treatment S.S. P.S.

EVOLUTION OF THE DISEASE

INVOLUTION OF THE DISEASE

HERING'S LAW

Accident, pain +++ = acute crisis: confront it directly
During the alarm phase, calming is most important.
In the adaptation and the chronic state phases, both systems
must be addressed to bring up the energy.

LEGEND:

Sympathetic system = S.S.

Parasympathetic system = P.S.

Balance of the S.S. and P.S.

Life cannot be sustained.

The Alarm Phase of the Stress Mechanism

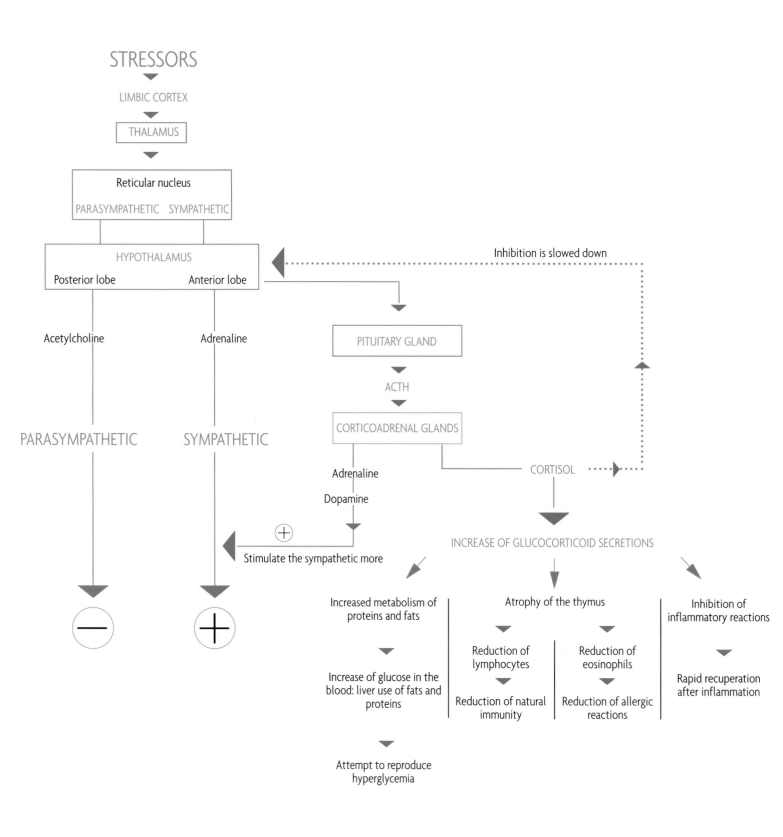

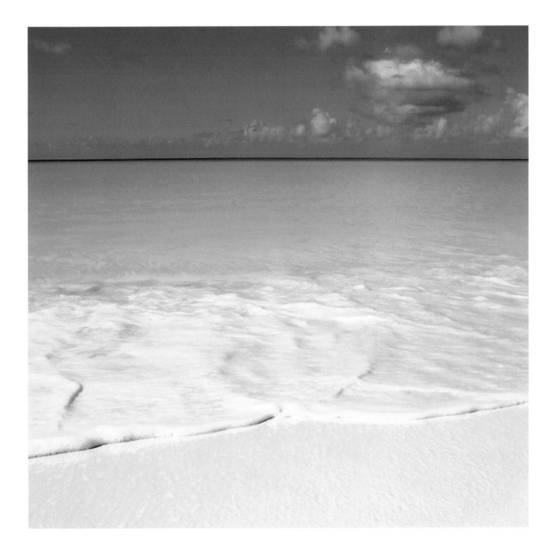

The Three Levels of Being

Reflexology acts globally on the three levels of being: physical, emotional or psychological, and mental. This concept of the human being's triple nature was passed down to us from Plato. I have retained this principle because of the lucid and clear analysis it allows us in understanding human behavior. However, let us not forget that these three terms, formerly body, soul, and spirit, are absolutely inextricable in reality. They can only seem independent; their autonomy is entirely relative because each one perpetually interacts with the others.

An emotional shock—for example, the news of the death of a close friend or relative—creates a state of imbalance in the body on the physical plane (tears, loss of energy, muscular fatigue, loss of appetite, and digestive dysfunction). A mental reaction will often come into play (reasonable analysis of the event, will to rise to the challenge at hand, decision to restore the rhythms of ordinary life), and in certain cases it can allow a return to psychic balance, then to the physical balance of the body—or vice versa.

These three levels of being are laid out on the feet in distinct regions.

The Physical Level, or "Tentorium Sacrum"

This level is located on the calcaneus and reflects the structure of the cells, the nerves, the chemical mediators, the fluids, and the tissues (fascias, organs, and so forth). Everything that makes up the physical body can be treated on the tentorium sacrum.

The tentorium sacrum includes the coccygeal plexus, connected with sexuality and reproduction, and the hypogastric plexus, connected to the adrenal glands. Treatment of the tentorium sacrum is performed on the reflex zones of the coccyx, the pubic rim, the iliopubic ramus, the ischiopubic ramus, the obturator foramen, and the sciatic spine.

The Emotional (or Psychic) Level, or "Tentorium Medium"

This tentorium is located in the mid-foot area, which is the reflex headquarters for the adrenal glands and numerous organs: the liver, stomach, spleen, pancreas, heart, lungs, and kidneys. It is the center for digestion, as well as a reservoir for emotions.

The tentorium medium includes the solar plexus, connected with the pancreas; the cardiac plexus, connected with the thymus; and the thyroid plexus, connected with the thyroid and the parathyroids. Treatment of the tentorium medium takes place on the reflex zones for the crura of the diaphragm, the rib insertions, and the diaphragm dome and, more important, on the reflex zones for the stomach, gastroesophageal sphincter, and heart. (See page 68.)

The Mental Level, or the "Tentorium Cerebelli"

This level is located on the toes. It contains the sense organs of sight, hearing, smell, and taste, which permit our perception of the outer world in part; the brain studies this data from the environment. The degree of perception and interpretation will vary depending upon the individual. The same is therefore true for the varied behaviors people have in response to a single event. In some therapies, the mental level is considered to be the highest priority.

The tentorium cerebelli includes the pituitary plexus, whose corresponding gland is the pituitary gland,

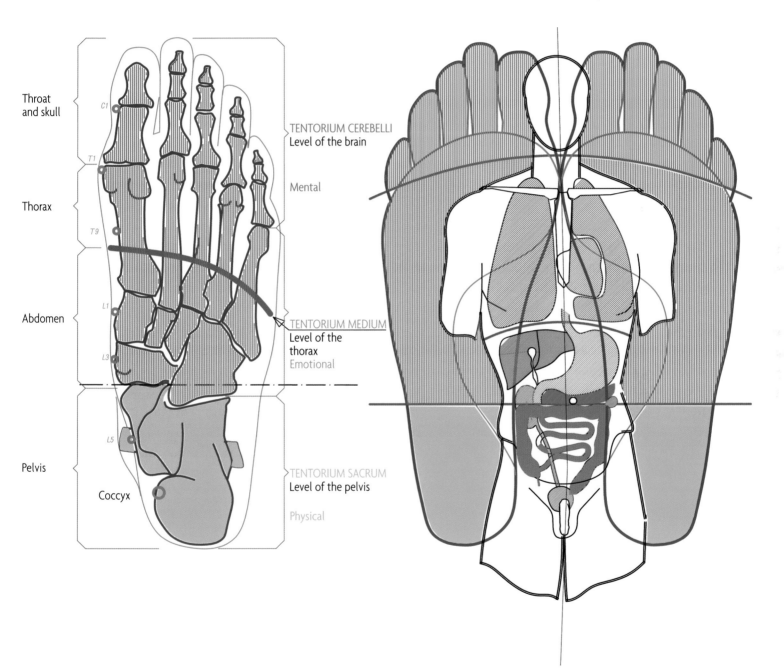

Throat
and skull

C1

TENTORIUM CEREBELLI
Level of the brain

Mental

Thorax

T1

T9

Abdomen

L1

L3

TENTORIUM MEDIUM
Level of the
thorax
Emotional

Pelvis

L5

TENTORIUM SACRUM
Level of the pelvis

Physical

Coccyx

and the pineal plexus, whose corresponding gland is the pineal gland. In addition to its own zones, treatment of the tentorium cerebelli is performed on the reflex zones of the sphenobasilar symphysis and the falx cerebri; on the zones of the periphery of the foramen magnum and the posterior foramen lacerum; and on the zones of the sphenofrontal, the occipitomastoidal, the temporomandibular, the lambdoidal, the coronal, and the parietosquamous sutures. (See pages 128 and 129.)

Treating the Three Levels of Being with Reflexology

Among the effects of reflexology treatment is the reduction of deep blockages that could potentially cause future health problems. The results provided by reflexology are even more valuable when viewed using the criteria offered by Hering's law.

The words spoken by the "other," especially when the other is the therapist, have unsuspected power. They can either help the healing process or create deep wounds. How a diagnosis is phrased, the way the treatment itself is described, and the terms used in a psychological exploration should be subject to the therapist's constant attention and prudence.

No treatment should be undertaken until the patient has received a thorough checkup and basic care to regulate the different systems of the body. The practitioner should first treat the cranial membranes (these are the dura mater, the arachnoid, the pia mater), then the cranial sutures, the cranial nerves, the plexuses, with treatment ending, depending on the case, with the cerebral or pelvic zones.

We will later see in greater detail, in the chapter "From Reflex to Consciousness," that the bits of information coming to us from our senses or brain wend their way in the form of electrical impulses; these impulses are born of the infinitesimal chemical exchanges that take place in our body on the molecular level. This information becomes imprinted in our body in the form of a hologram, shared by all the different parts of the body at the same moment. The interdependent sharing of a sensation, a thought, or an action occurs on a scale where all distinctions among the physical, mental, and emotional disappear.

From here, far from restricting ourselves to a diagnostic process perfected by a medical philosophy approaching pathological conditions from a strictly somatic angle, we must now agree to take the whole of the human being into account. What's needed now to put the appropriate treatment methods to work is to draw specifically from the resources of an emotional, mental, and spiritual nature that are present in the individual.

The body is a marvelous tool, endowed by nature with all kinds of protective mechanisms. A great many negative factors are required to throw it out of order. But there are times when only one is needed to bring about profound illness, simply because it carries with it a large enough emotional discharge—from something experienced in isolation and impossible to verbalize.

Hering's Law
Hierarchy of the Symptoms of the Three Levels

Mental Plane

Total mental confusion
Destructive ideas
Paranoiac delusions
Delirium; hallucinations
Lethargy
Slow reactions
Sluggish and absent mind
Lack of concentration
Forgetfulness and carelessness

Emotional Body

Suicidal depression
Apathy
Sadness
Anger
Phobias
Anxiety
Irritability
Lack of satisfaction

Physical Body

Brain disorders
Heart trouble
Liver problems
Endocrine system problems
Pulmonary disorders
Renal disorders
Bone problems
Muscular problems
Skin problems

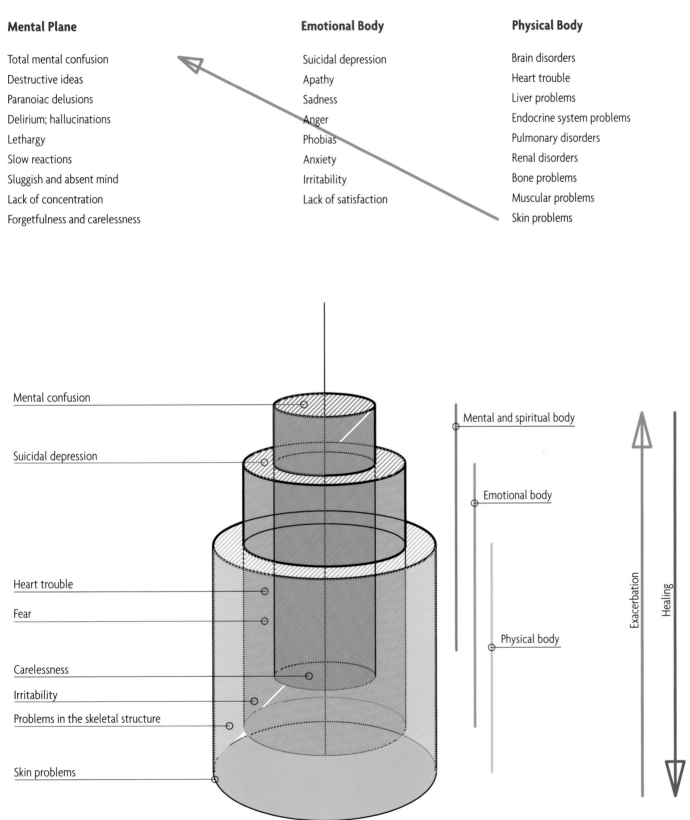

The Three Levels of Being

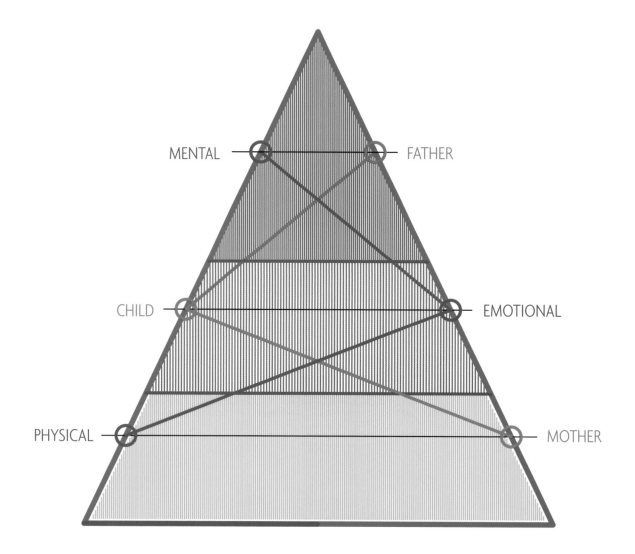

148 ◆ Total Reflexology Therapy

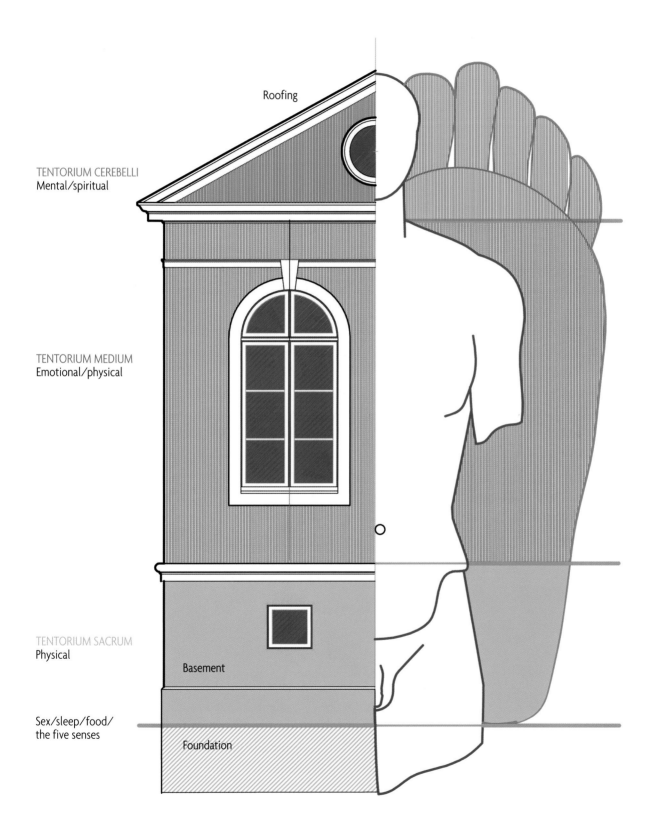

Roofing

TENTORIUM CEREBELLI
Mental/spiritual

TENTORIUM MEDIUM
Emotional/physical

TENTORIUM SACRUM
Physical

Basement

Sex/sleep/food/
the five senses

Foundation

From Reflex to Consciousness

In the brain, information circulates from one neuron to the next in the form of electrical impulses. The number of neurons our brain contains is around a hundred billion. Their collective activity ensures our relationship to the outside world, to our emotions, and to our actions. Together, they form a complex web in which a single neuron can be in direct connection with hundreds of thousands of others.

Neurons are organized into groups that are specialized in performing different tasks. The information they transmit is dealt with, depending on the nature of the information, in a good many regions of the brain simultaneously. The messages circulating within these "associative" regions contain data that can be just as easily visual or olfactory as tactile or related to motor function. The associative zones play a crucial role in higher mental functions, such as memory or language. These mental functions bring each of the vast regions of the cerebral cortex into play. In these zones, which are both motor and sensorial, numerous operations are performed that allow perception to be linked to the control of movement.

Unlike a computer, which responds to outside signals in a passive manner, *the brain is an autonomous instrument capable of organizing its own activity.*

How Do Neurons Function?

Information is transmitted from one neuron to the next by a neurotransmitter, a chemical messenger that triggers an electrical signal by binding to its "receptor." Recent studies have shown that in certain situation, the glial cells of the nervous system manufacture an enzyme that synthesizes nitric oxide, which amplifies the efficiency of transmissions among neurons and plays an essential role in the process of memorization and learning new skills.

The brain does not act alone. The spinal cord, effectively an extension of the brain, is a channel formed of nervous tissue roughly as thick as the little finger and around sixty centimeters in length. With the brain, it forms the central nervous system.

Along the entire length of the spinal cord, there are thirty-one pairs of nerves entering and leaving at regular intervals, forming the peripheral nervous system. Each pair connects the spinal cord to a specific region of the body. The nervous fibers entering the spinal cord (sensory fibers) convey the sensations sent from a given region, and the fibers leaving the spinal cord (motor fibers) carry the commands to the muscles of the same region. The nerves, bundles of nervous fibers that are extensions of the neurons, therefore play a dual role. They convey the sensorial messages coming from the sense organs (the skin, eyes, ears, nose, and mouth) and command the muscles.

Consciousness

The most extraordinary power human beings have at their disposal to triumph over disease is their own consciousness. But what is consciousness? How does it work? How can the body produce something on the order of the mind? Does it categorize as purely biological? Or is it in the category of purely mental phenomena? In this case, by what subtle mechanisms does our nonmaterial thought command the movements of our physical body?

During the eighteenth century, Descartes imagined that the mind and body interacted through the intermediary of the pineal gland. Spinoza believed that they formed one sole entity considered from two different points of view. Consciousness would therefore become the mental expression of a real physical event.

Confirming the latter theory, in *Descartes' Error*, Antonio Damasio investigates the biological mechanisms at play in the manufacturing of an emotion or feeling. This is all well and good, but one question still remains: What mechanisms, of what order and what nature, allow for the transition from the emotion or sensation felt to the awareness of the self feeling that emotion or sensation? In the space defined by the two terms of this proposition, we have installed the concept of consciousness as the fundamental ability *to think ourselves.*

Damasio shows that this mechanism, as complex as it may be, falls outside the jurisdiction of the "mind." In fact, patients afflicted with various disorders affecting their reasoning, their ability to think coherently, or their ability to handle sensorial information do not lose awareness of themselves.

On the other hand, when the awareness of self is disrupted, all the intellectual and emotional operations performed by the mind suffer. Consciousness therefore appears to be the fundamental base, essential for all actions involving the will; impossible to grasp in itself, it is the process that conditions all the others.

For Antonio Damasio, what explains the appearance of consciousness in the evolution of living beings is the functioning of a central system that constantly presides over the proper functioning of the entire body. It is here that Damasio's reasoning again meets Spinoza's intuition. "Consciousness," he says, "is nothing other than the cartography that the mind makes of the state of the alterations in the body. Consciousness is produced when the brain's devices of representation engender an explanation in non-verbal images of the way the body's own state is affected."

Consciousness, as the "very feeling of self," results in reality from complex programs put together by the body to harmonize the totality of corporeal mechanisms and to maintain its life—at every moment. Under this aspect, the "very feeling of self" appears as the sole face that emerges from the mechanisms of consciousness.

From Reflex to Consciousness

Echoing the theories of wave mechanics and electromagnetism, or the theories on the constitution of matter from the scale of the atom to the scale of the universe, and beyond the assumptions of biology proper, the study of the bioenergy of human beings and their rhythms and the analysis of their vibratory manifestations have made us comfortable today with the idea that we are only a particular expression in space and time of this very universe—as long as there's proof that we answer to the same laws.

Every strand of DNA contains the entire program for a human, animal, or plant—which, fully developed, will be several billion times bigger than this strand, and whose innermost cell will in its turn contain the entire program for the species. Seeing ourselves on the infinitesimal scale of being human, as "a point between two infinities," as Pascal saw us, could it be that our consciousness is to the laws of the universe—the laws on which the equilibrium of the universe depends—what a single strand of DNA is to the entire human race? Couldn't consciousness be an emanation on the scale—an emanation divided infinitely but infinitely complex and powerful—of the universal law, of "universal consciousness"?

If the answer is yes, these words by Socrates now resonate fully with a great burst of truth: "Know thyself and thou shalt know the universe and its gods."

Therefore, every fiber of our being contains a portion of our consciousness and consequently reacts in alignment with that consciousness. Conversely, we can act at a distance, through thought, on every part of our body. A positive thought can act in a positive way on all or part of the body. Conversely, a negative thought can seriously compromise our health, even when it does not attach itself to the physical body. Hatred destroys the one who hates.

Far from being simply a moralistic notion, the state

of love is the very state of health. Love of nature, love of beauty, love of life, love of others, love of self—all bring serenity, harmony, and balance down to the very tiniest cell of our thinking, feeling, acting being. Furthermore, the sacred is not exclusive to religion; it is all around us, in the joy of a child and in the beauty of a tree. Let us respect it. The sacred is also within us: Let us also respect ourselves.

As discussed in the chapter on the craniosacral system, brain function is triggered by the perception of sound waves and electromagnetic waves translated into electrical impulses. The CSF transmits electromagnetic information, which it retains in memory, to the entire body via the spinal cord. Consequently, the information originating from our cells and shared, as vibrations, by all the parts of the brain is in return simultaneously shared by all parts of the body.

Between the infinite smallness of the "thinking" world of DNA and the infinite largeness of universal consciousness, couldn't it be said that on our scale of existence, there is in fact a single memory and a single brain—those of the whole of humanity? And wouldn't it follow that each time someone increases his or her clarity of thought, harmony of feelings, or beauty of actions, it is a holographic present given to the whole of humanity?

Quantum physics explains that on the level of atomic observation, reality is altered by the observer. In the same way, in medicine we are noting that the patient's state of mind can affect his or her power to recuperate in unfathomable ways. Perhaps reflex and consciousness are different only by the scale of time and space used to measure them.

The pianist Glenn Gould said: "The goal of art is to gradually attain, over the course of a lifetime, a state of wonderment."

Let us not stop aspiring to reach this state.

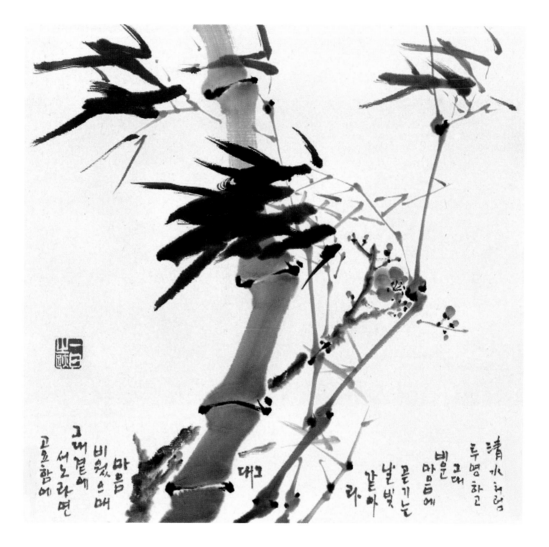

대고

맑은 마음에
끊기는 날빛
같아라

마음 비웠으매
그대 붓에 써노라면
고요함이

清水처럼
투명하고
그대

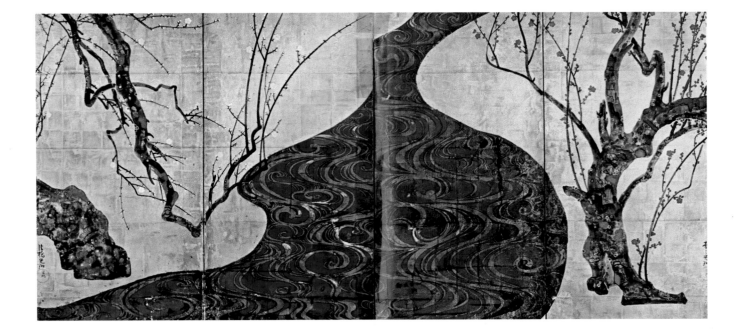

About the Author

During the course of her medical studies at the University of London, where she specialized in osteopathy, Dr. Martine Faure-Alderson became aware that beyond all the various medical disciplines, one constant held sway: The human being is a whole. After this realization, she concentrated her studies on natural and alternative therapies. For a period of twenty-five years she studied naturopathy, acupuncture, phytotherapy, and homeopathy in England and in South America.

During the 1960s, she discovered reflexology with Doreen Bayly, a student of Eunice Ingham. At this time, Dr. Faure-Alderson was working in a clinic where several of her patients were experiencing digestive problems. She began treating the zones on their feet that correspond with the digestive system. A three-month trial period was sufficient to demonstrate the effectiveness of this treatment. Inspired by these results, she conducted specific clinical research with Doreen Bayly.

In 1968, Dr. Faure-Alderson began teaching reflexology at seminars. Until that time, reflexology had been legitimated only through empirical evidence, but her medical training allowed her to articulate in scientific terms the workings of reflexology. She brought in the precision required to locate the exact points or zones on the foot that correspond to the particular organs or regions of the body. This same scientific rigor informs her diagnoses and the "reflex treatment" she uses to address the pathologies of her patients.

Inspired by the holistic approach she applies to understanding her patient (his particular makeup and prior physical, mental, or psychological history), as well as to diagnosis and treatment, she named her school Total Reflexology Therapy.

During the 1970s, Dr. Faure-Alderson advanced Total Reflexology Therapy by integrating the idea of stress syndrome, as revealed by Selye's research, and the importance of the occipital zones, whose reactions confirm the reflexes of the sole of the foot. During the 1990s, after researching with her students, she gave her teaching the finishing touch with the incorporation of the effects of craniosacral therapy on foot reflexology. Her research is now focused on the primary respiratory mechanism, the cerebrospinal fluid, the cranial nerves, and the three levels of being (physical, emotional, mental).

Gradually, thanks to the insights gained from her practice, she incorporated other modalities, such as naturopathy, homeopathy, and acupuncture, into her work and practice, thereby creating a synthesis of all the natural therapies and giving Total Reflexology Therapy solid multidisciplinary foundations. Foot reflexology as practiced in Total Reflexology Therapy is truly a holistic therapy.

Today Dr. Martine Faure-Alderson teaches and gives conferences throughout the world, including in the United States, Canada, Australia, New Zealand, and Europe.

Total Reflexology Training Seminars

Although this book was originally published in French, the author offers training in Total Reflexology Therapy in English. English-speaking practitioners and other interested parties can contact the Craniosacral Reflexology Institute for information on the training seminars provided there.

www.craniosacralreflexologyinstitute.com

A two-year course of study in Total Reflexology Therapy is available to French speakers. The first year is devoted to the study or complete review of anatomy, physiology, and applied pathology. The second year is open directly to health professionals and devoted to training in reflexology proper. Those successfully passing the two-year course will receive a certificate. The program is supplemented by postgraduate seminars in natural medicines, puberty and menopause, the cran-iosacral system, the three levels of being, the immune system, and the emotional body in reflexology.

Interested students may contact Dr. Martine Faure-Alderson at:

Website: www.craniosacralreflexologyinstitute.com
E-mail: martinefa@craniosacralreflexologyinstitute.com

For those wishing to contact her on other business:
      Website: www.natclinicrem.co.uk
      (short for "natural clinic remedy")
      E-mail: info@natclinicrem.co.uk

French speakers can contact Martine Faure-Alderson at:
      Website: www.rttfa.com
      e-mail: info@rttfa.com

Acknowledgments

I would like to offer my warmest thanks to my two most valuable collaborators, Antoinette Conejero Llopart and Noëlle Jongit, without whom this book would never have seen the light of day.

Thanks as well to Josette Mort for her dedicated and fastidious work.

Special thanks to the Curie Institute in Paris, which was the first to give a favorable reception to our research by accepting the fact that foot reflexology holds an essential place among all the disciplines offering support to its patients.

And finally, for the similar welcome they gave me to their institutions of health care and research, thanks to the following:

Dr. Gwen Wyatt of Michigan State University

Mr. David Oliver of Sir Charles Gairdner Hospital in Perth, Australia

Mrs. Kim Krusten of Sydney Adventist Hospital in Sydney, Australia

Mrs. Eyglo Benediktsdottir of the Landspitali University Hospital in Reykjavik, Iceland

Bibliography

Barral, Jean-Pierre. *Visceral Manipulation.* Vol. II. Rev. ed. Seattle: Eastland Press, 2007. First English-language ed. 1989. First published as *Manipulations viscérales,* vol. II, in 1987 by Maloine Éditions, Paris.

Barral, Jean-Pierre, and Pierre Mercier. *Visceral Manipulation.* Vol. I. Rev. ed. Seattle: Eastland Press, 2006. First English-language ed. 1988. First published as *Manipulations viscérales,* vol. I, by Maloine Éditions, Paris.

Batmanghelidj, Fereydoon. *Your Body's Many Cries for Water: You Are Not Sick, You Are Thirsty!* Falls Church, Va.: Global Health Solutions, 1995.

Brouillet, Denis, and Arielle Syssau. *La maladie d'Alzheimer: Mémoire et vieillissement.* [Alzheimer's Disease: Memory and Aging.] Paris: PUF, Éditions Que Sais-Je?, 2005.

Carter, Rita. *Mapping the Mind.* London: Phoenix, 1988.

Chia, Mantak. *Awaken Healing Energy through the Tao.* Santa Fe: Aurora Press, 1983.

Childre, Doc Lew, and Martin Howard. *The Heartmath Solution.* New York: HarperCollins, 1999.

Chopra, Deepak. *Life after Death: The Burden of Proof.* New York: Harmony, 2006.

Davidson, John. *The Web of Life.* Oxford, U.K.: C. W. Daniels, 1988.

De Mello, Anthony. *Awareness.* New York: Doubleday, 1990.

Goleman, Daniel. *Emotional Intelligence: Why It Can Matter More Than IQ.* New York: Bantam Books, 1995.

Guillain, France. *Les bains dérivatifs.* [Derivative Baths.] Saint-Julien-en-Genevois: Éditions Jouvence, 1995.

Guo, Bisong, and Andrew Powell. *Listen to Your Body: The Wisdom of the Dao.* Honolulu: University of Hawaii Press, 2001.

Israel, Luciën. *Cerveau droit, cerveau gauche: cultures et civilisations.* [Right Brain, Left Brain: Cultures and Civilizations.] Paris: Éditions Plon, 1995.

Issartel, Lionelle, and Marielle Issartel. *L'Ostéopathie exactement.* [Osteopathy Exactly.] Paris: Éditions Robert Laffont, 1983.

Janet, Jacques. *La médecine bio dynamique.* [Biodynamic Medicine.] Paris: Éditions R. Jollois, 1999.

Julian, O. A. *Materia Medica of New Homeopathic Remedies.* Beaconsfield, U.K.: Beaconsfield Publishers, 1984.

Kieffer, Daniel. *L'Homme empoisonné: Cures végétales pour libérer son corps et son esprit.* [The Poisoned Man: Plant-Based Cures to Liberate His Body and Mind.] Paris: Éditions Grancher, 1993.

Kübler-Ross, Elisabeth. *The Wheel of Life: A Memoir of Living and Dying.* New York: Scribners, 1997.

Labonté, Marie Lise. *Se guérir autrement, c'est possible: Comment j'ai vaincu ma maladie.* [Another Way to Heal Yourself Is Possible: How I Conquered My Disease.] Quebec City: Les Éditions de l'Homme, 2001.

Magoun, Harold Ives. *Osteopathy in the Cranial Field,* 3rd edition. Kirksville, Mo.: Journal Print Co., 1976.

Netter, Frank H. *Atlas of Human Anatomy.* 4th ed. Philadelphia: Saunders, 2006.

Nkaye, Emiléa. *Le vieillissement: Une approche psychosomatique.* [Aging: A Psychosomatic Approach.] Paris: Éditions L'Harmattan, 2000.

Rueff, Dominique. *Hormones végétales naturelles aujourd'hui: Andropause, menopause—des solutions* naturelles et sans risque. [Natural Plant-Based Hormones Today: Andropause, Menopause—Natural Solutions without Risk.] Saint-Julien-en-Genevois, Switzerland: Éditions Jouvence, 1997.

Seignalet, Jean. L'Alimentation ou la troisième médecine. [Nutrition or the Third Medicine.] Paris: Éditions Francois-Xavier de Guibert, 2004.

Selawry, Alla. Types fonctionnels métalliques en psychologie et médecine. [Functional Metallic Types in Psychology and Medicine.] Paris: Guy Trédaniel Éditeur, 1990.

Servan-Schreiber, David. Guérir le stress, l'anxiété et la dépression sans medicaments ni psychanalyse. [Healing Stress, Anxiety and Depression without Medication or Psychoanalysis.] Paris: Éditions Robert Laffont, 2003.

Thomasson, Nitza. Le Vieillissement cérébral. [Cerebral Aging.] Paris: PUF, Éditions Que Sais-Je?, 2000.

Upledger, John E. A Brain Is Born: Exploring the Birth and Development of the Central Nervous System. Berkeley, Calif.: North Atlantic Books, 1996.

———. Your Inner Physician and You. Palm Beach Gardens, Fla.: UI Enterprises and Berkeley, Calif.: North Atlantic Books, 1997.

Upledger, John E., and Jon D. Vredevoogd. Craniosacral Therapy. Seattle: Eastland Press, 1983.

Véret, Patrick, and Yvonne Parquer. Traité de Nutripuncture: physiologie, information cellulaire. [Treatise on Nutripuncture: Physiology, Cellular Information.] Méolans-Revel: Éditions DésIris, 2005.

List of Plates

Index

reflex points, 128–29
superior cervical ganglion, 137

dairy products, 62
Damasio, Antonio, 151
depression, 40, 76, 100, 109, 112
dermatomes, 32, 33
diabetes, 38, 109
diet
    aging and, 88
    eating correctly, 94
    immune system and, 76
    preventive nutrition, 106–7
    skeletal system and, 52
digestive system
    described, 56–57
    fiber for, 107
    reflex points/zones, 57, 68, 69
    solar (digestive) plexus, 36
    water needed by, 110
dispnea, 94
DNA (deoxyribonucleic acid), 18–19,
    21, 151

ectoderm, 22, 24
ectomorph, 28–29
edema, 38, 70
elderly persons, 13, 15, 74, 88–89
electromagnetic energy, 84, 152
elimination, 6, 94, 102
embryo, 22, 23–24
emotional (or psychic) level of being,
    36, 144, 145
emotions
    brain function affected by, 20
    bringing back to consciousness, 102
    emotional quotient (EQ), 100
    emotional shock, 102
    felt in the stomach, 62
    heart as site for, 98
    love, 151–52
    negative, 100, 112
    positive, 100
    reflex points/zones, 130–32
    relationship between heart and brain,
        99
    repressed, 16

endocrine glands, 40–43
endoderm, 22, 25
endomorph, 28, 29
endorphins, 112, 114
enzymes, 18
estrogen, 42–43
evolution, 19–20
exercise, 93, 94

fascia, 100, 102
fatigue, 76, 94, 109, 112
fear and anxiety, 15–16, 59, 62, 100,
    139
fever, 76, 81, 93
fiber, 107
fibrosis, 29
Fitzgerald, William, 2
foot
    arch of, 9, 55
    bones of, 8–9
    clinical aspect, 12
    See also reflex points/zones
forces of life, 84–85
Frymann, Viola, 122
functional and structural types, 29

Gardner, Howard, 100
gastric pains, 109, 110
glucagon, 42, 44, 76
Goleman, Daniel, 100
grooming and hygiene, 94
growth hormone, 44, 48
Guille, Etienne, 20
gut-associated lymphoid tissue (GALT),
    74
gymnastics, neuronal, 88

habits, reprogramming, 16
Hamer, Ryke Geerd, 20
headaches/migraines, 110, 112, 122
heart
    about, 98
    cardiac coherence and cerebral
        harmony, 101
    cardiac plexus, 36
    communicating with the brain, 98–99
    electromagnetic field of, 84

intelligence of, 98, 100
    reflex points/zones, 63, 67
heartbeat, 84
heartburn, 110
heart disease, 29
Hering's Law, 5, 102, 139–40, 146
hiatal hernia, 110
hippocampus, 87, 88, 124
history of reflexology, 2
hologram, 20, 146, 152
homeopathy, 81
horizontal occipital zones, 120, 121
hormones
    described, 40
    emotions and, 139
    reflex points/zones, 45, 68
    sleep and, 47, 48
    synthesis with plexuses, 68
    See also specific hormones
hygiene and grooming, 94
hyperacidity, 106
hyperkeratosis, 12
hypogastric plexus, 36
hypoglycemia, 38, 44
hypothalamus, 6, 40–41, 42, 47

illness
    first stage of, 81
    manifesting in reflex zones, 7
    symptoms, 6, 102
immune system
    evaluating, 70
    fluidic interrelations, 76
    overview, 74
    stimulating, 38
    stress and, 40
    thymus and, 42
infertility, 15
Ingham, Eunice, 2
insomnia, 15, 100
insulin, 42, 44, 48, 106, 114
intelligence quotient (IQ), 100
intestines, 76, 94

kidneys, 59, 106, 110
kidney stones, 29
Kirlian photography, 20

skin tone, 12
skull
    described, 122
    occipital palpation, 13
    occipital zones, 5, 13, 120–21
sleep
    about, 47, 96
    disorders/insomnia, 15, 76, 96,
        100
    growth hormone and, 44, 48
    rapid eye movement (REM), 47–48,
        96
social welfare, 105
sodas, 109–10
solar (digestive) plexus, 36
spinal column, 41, 54, 150
spleen, 74, 76
stomach, 56
stress syndrome
    ACTH and, 44
    aging and, 88
    alarm phase of, 139, 142
    becoming conscious of, 76
    biotypes and, 29
    cardiac plexus affected by, 36
    dealing with, 6, 139–40
    immune system and, 40, 76
    nervous system affected by, 6
    reflex points/zones, 140
    six stages of, 139, 141
    stressors and stimuli, 138–39
    sympathetic nervous system and,
        139
    water used during, 112
structural and functional types, 29

subconscious, 102
superior cervical ganglion, 137
Sutherland, William, 122
sympathetic nervous system
    described, 6, 30
    distribution of, 31
    function of, 32
    stress' effect on, 139
sympathicontonic state, 76
symptoms, resurgence of, 6, 102
systems of the body, 50

T cells, 76
tea, 109–10, 114
testicles, 43, 60–61
testosterone, 43
third eye, 40
thought, negative, 112, 151
three levels of being, 36, 38, 144–46
thumbs, 34
thymus, 42, 74, 88
thyroid gland, 41–42
thyroid plexus, 36
thyroid-stimulating hormone (TSH),
    44, 48
toes, 34, 89, 124, 145
Total Reflexology Therapy
    contraindications for, 13
    described, 6
    end of the session, 13
    evaluating patient's biotype, 28
    evaluating the immune system, 70
    example of a treatment, obesity,
        15–16
    indications, 14

length of session, 13
observing the patient, 12–13
technique, 13
unconscious memories coming up,
    102
See also reflexology; reflex points/
    zones
toxins, 88
trauma, 15, 16, 20, 122, 124
tumors, 20, 112–13, 114

ulcers, 110
Upledger, John, 102
urinary system, 58–61
uterus, 60–61

vagus nerve, 98, 126
vasopressin, 116
vertical occipital zones, 120–21
vibrational fields, 20
vital force, 81–83
vitamins, 52, 88, 106, 107

water
    cerebral activity and, 114, 116
    coccygeal plexus ruled by, 36
    as medicine, 93–94
    pathological conditions due to
        dehydration, 112, 114, 116
    role in metabolism, 109–10
weight loss, 76
World Health Organization (WHO),
    105

yin and yang, 93, 94

Books of Related Interest

The Reflexology Manual
An Easy-to-Use Illustrated Guide to the Healing Zones
of the Hands and Feet
by Pauline Wills

Sexual Reflexology
Activating the Taoist Points of Love
by Mantak Chia and William U. Wei

The Reflexology Atlas
by Bernard C. Kolster, M.D., and Astrid Waskowiak, M.D.

Facial Reflexology
A Self-Care Manual
by Marie-France Muller, M.D., N.D., Ph.D.

Right Brain/Left Brain Reflexology
by Madeleine Turgeon, N.D.

Reflexology Today
The Stimulation of the Body's Healing Forces
through Foot Massage
by Doreen E. Bayly

Gemstone Reflexology
by Nora Kircher

The Acupressure Atlas
by Bernard C. Kolster, M.D., and Astrid Waskowiak, M.D.

INNER TRADITIONS • BEAR & COMPANY
P.O. Box 388
Rochester, VT 05767
1-800-246-8648
www.InnerTraditions.com

Or contact your local bookseller